Australian
FIRST AID

Australian
FIRST AID

Second Edition

VOLUME ONE

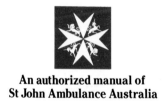

**An authorized manual of
St John Ambulance Australia**

St John Ambulance Australia
Canberra Avenue
Forrest ACT 2603

First edition 1984
Reprinted with corrections 1984-1988
Second edition completely rewritten 1989
Reprinted with corrections 2/1990, 4/1990, 7/1990, 10/1990,
1/1991, 4/1991, 6/1991, 9/1991, 12/1991, 3/1992
6/1992, 9/1992, 12/1992

Australian first aid volume one
    Includes index

    ISBN 0 949569 17 8 (Vol. 1)
    ISBN 0 949569 16 X (Set)

Editors: Lynne Macdonald, Alison Verhoeven
Designer: Pauline McClenahan, Bookworks
Illustrator: Heather Strahan
Production management: Russell G. Gilbert Pty. Ltd., John Cook
Typeset in Cheltenham Light by Savage Type Pty. Ltd. (Brisbane)
Reproduction by Enticott (Melbourne)
Printed by Canberra Press (Melb.) Pty. Ltd.
Bound by M & M Binders Pty. Ltd. (Melbourne)

Contents

Acknowledgments

St John Ambulance Australia would like to thank all those who have contributed to the development of the Australian First Aid project. In particular, the organization thanks the following groups and individuals for their support.

St John Ambulance Australia Centres in all states

Members of the St John Ambulance Australia Operations Branch in the ACT, and particularly Mandy and Phillip Langdon, for assistance with the preparation of illustrations

Members of the Curriculum Committee — Dr Edward Brentnall, Dr Barry Collins, Megan Holmes, Peter McMurtrie, Elaine Ondaatje, Nancy Sly

Members of the Technical Advisory Committee — Dr Brian Ancell, Mr Allan Beech, Dr Brian Purssey

Staff of the National Headquarters, and especially Janita Hopkins and Mary Maxwell for typing the manuscript

Australia and New Zealand Burn Association

Alcohol and Drug Foundation

Asthma Foundation of NSW

Diabetes Australia (NSW)

Epilepsy Association of Australia

Institute of Ambulance Officers (Australia)

Royal Australasian College of Surgeons — Faculty of Anaesthetists

Sir George Bedbrook; Sgt Brian Carr; Mark Compton; Dr Louis Fenelon; Dr Peter Fenner; Graham Morrow; Dr Harry Oxer; Professor John Pearn; Dr K.C. Wan; Dr Jeff Wassertheil; Dr John Williamson

Foreword

First aid remains one of the most important of all life's skills. The simple yet essential skills to preserve life in an emergency, to protect a casualty and to hasten the healing of wounds, are skills which no parent, partner, motorist or workmate can do without. Acute illness and sudden injury have no respect for age or status, or place or time. It is thus one of the imperatives of modern living to 'do the right thing' by those around us. *Australian First Aid* is one vehicle by which these important skills can be achieved.

Australian First Aid has for several years been an Australian best seller. It is the major resource for the teaching of first aid to the Australian public. Tailored for Australian conditions, it has a special relevance for all those who wish to acquire these essential skills.

This current text is continually modified and updated as new conditions occur. The text is thus topical and relevant, and is one of the cheapest forms of insurance to help save life, to protect casualties, and to hasten the convalescence of the sick and injured.

This book has been divided into two parts for easier handling. Volume 1 comprises chapters 1 to 19 and is designed to accompany the St John Ambulance Australia Senior First Aid course. It provides information for emergency first aid and the management of common injuries and illnesses. Volume 2 comprises chapters 20 to 31 and contains advanced and specialist information.

First aid is a practical subject. The approach to helping the victims of injury and illness depends on a firm practical foundation of being able to make a diagnosis, and to commence management as a true 'hands-on' skill. This book will take you through these points, together with a minimal theoretical component, to help you understand what you are doing. The steps in management of a wide variety of important illnesses and injuries have been simplified in this text, and every attempt has been made to ensure that the subject material is relevant to everyday life.

Australia is well supplied with emergency services. However, the great size of the country makes it impossible for those services to be available in all circumstances, and at all times and in all places. St John Ambulance Australia believes that this text will provide you with the information that will be useful in the widest variety of real life circumstances that you may encounter.

While the text sets out in detail the steps in diagnosis and management, it is no substitute for a practical first aid course. Participation in such a course will give you the confidence, as well as the experience, to become fully proficient and skilled in the management of the ill and injured.

Professor John Pearn
Director of Training

Illustrations

Introduction

What is first aid?

- the initial care of the ill or injured.

The aims of first aid

First aid aims to:
- promote a safe environment
- preserve life
- prevent injury or illness from becoming worse
- help promote recovery
- protect the unconscious
- reassure the ill or injured.

The first aider aims to prevent:
- further danger to himself, others or the casualty
- the casualty dying
- the casualty's condition becoming worse
- delay in the casualty's recovery
- any harmful intervention.

What is medical aid?

- treatment by a doctor, registered nurse or ambulance officer.

First aid begins when the first aider arrives at the scene of an incident, and continues until the casualty recovers, or medical aid arrives. The first aider may be required to remain and assist.

How to seek medical aid

If possible, send someone else to seek medical aid immediately. Do not leave the casualty. However, if you are alone at the scene of an incident, and it is unlikely that anyone will arrive for some time, you will need to leave the casualty and seek help as soon as possible.

Messages should be brief. You should confirm that they are understood. State your telephone number, the exact place with directions, the time and nature of the incident. Give the number of casualties with an indication of their condition. Ask the likely time of arrival of aid.

Describe location

Name of district, suburb, etc: ..... *NUNAWADING* .....

Name of street, road, highway, etc: ..... *Maroondah Hwy* .....

Nearest cross street (suburban): ..... *Springvale Road* .....

Distance from town or major landmark (country) ..... kms

North ☐   South ☐   East ☐   West ☐

of .... (describe town or landmark)

Give accident details

Number of people hurt ..... *3 (2 adults, 1 infant)* .....

Time of accident (if known) ..... *3.15 am approx* .....

Time this message written ..... *3.21 am* .....

Notes *Truck and family sedan have collided on corner — Big petrol spill. Infant critical. Melway 48 F9 (1984)*

.....

0.1 How to seek medical aid

1

What a first aider uses

First aid kits

Bandages

Slings

First aid kits

Your first aid kit contains items such as:
- bandages
- dressings
- slings
- scissors
- safety pins.

However, you will sometimes have to use whatever material you can find.

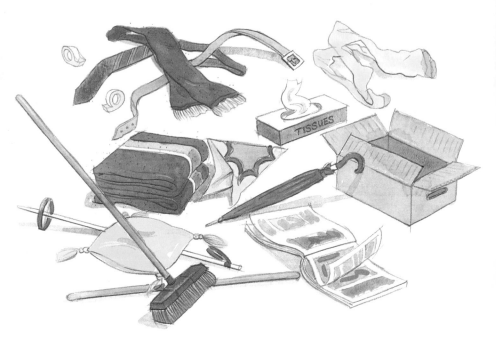

1.1 Improvized materials for first aid

Bandages

These are used to:
- control bleeding
- keep dressings in position
- give support and pain relief
- restrict movement
- immobilize fractures, usually with the aid of splints.

Dressings

Dressings should be:
- sterile or clean
- non-stick.

They may be made from a single square of clean cloth. They are used to:
- control bleeding
- protect wounds
- minimize swelling
- prevent infection
- ease pain.

Pads

Pads are applied over a dressing for direct pressure. A folded triangular bandage may be used.

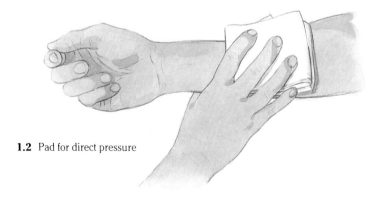

1.2 Pad for direct pressure

Triangular bandages

Triangular bandages can be used as dressings, pads, padding or slings. If used to bandage a wound, they should be secured with a reef knot. They can be made by cutting a one metre square piece of cloth into two diagonal pieces. To fold a triangular bandage as a pad:

☐ fold in half, i.e. point to base

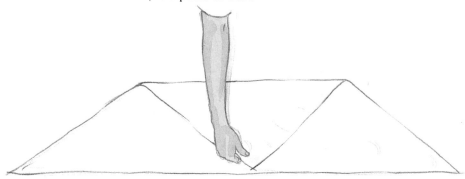

☐ fold in half again to make a broad bandage

☐ fold in half again to make a narrow bandage

☐ fold ends to middle

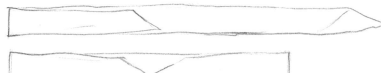

☐ repeat

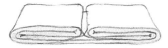

☐ fold what is left in half to make a pad. This may be easily packed away in your first aid kit.

1.3 Folding a triangular bandage

Roller bandages

These are made from long strips of material and come in different widths. They can be used to make a simple spiral for use on parts of the body that are fairly straight, such as the wrist or fingers:

☐ begin with the head of the bandage facing upwards and the tail pointing in towards the casualty

1.4 a

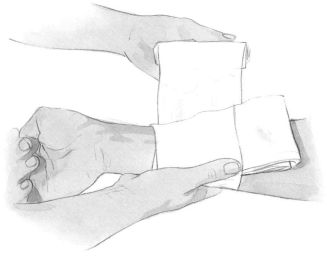

☐ carry the bandage around the limb in a spiral pattern

b

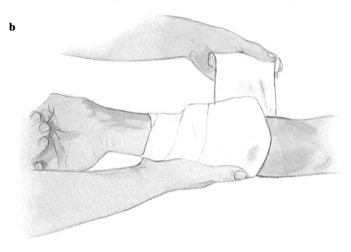

☐ each turn of the bandage covers two-thirds of the one before it and the edges should be kept parallel. Fasten the end with a safety pin, adhesive tape, or tuck in.

c

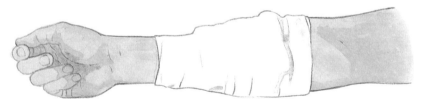

1.4 a-c Applying a roller bandage

The reef knot

Use a reef knot to secure bandages and slings because:
- it will not come undone easily by itself
- it is flat and will not dig into wounds
- it is easily undone by anyone managing the casualty.

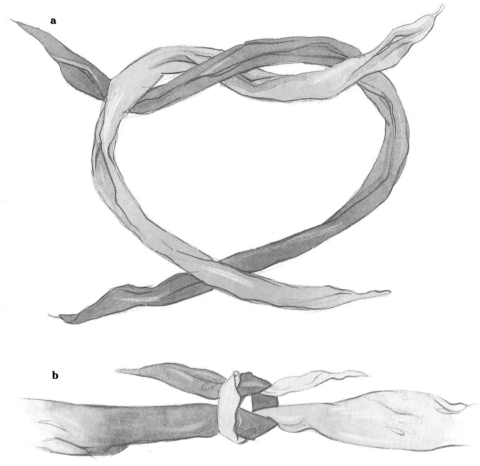

1.5 a-b Tying a reef knot

The clove hitch

This is used to make a collar and cuff sling:
- ☐ make two loops — one towards you, the other away from you. Place your fingers under the loops and bring them together
- ☐ slide the loops over your arm with the loose ends together.

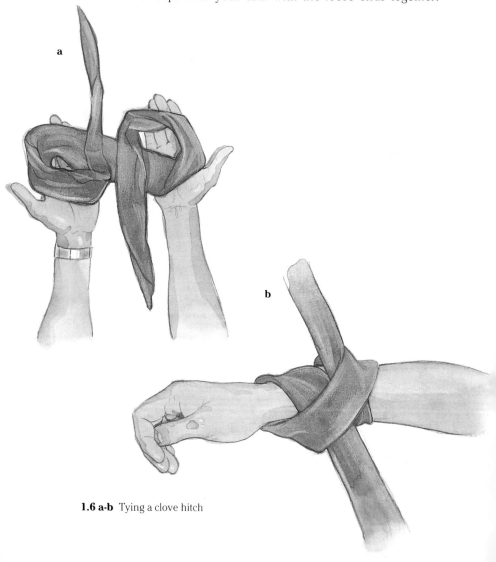

1.6 a-b Tying a clove hitch

The collar and cuff sling

This is useful for the casualty with a fracture of the upper arm or an injured hand:

- □ make a clove hitch, using a narrow bandage
- □ put the loops over the wrist of the injured arm
- □ gently elevate the injured arm against the casualty's chest
- □ tie the bandage ends together around the neck using a reef knot.

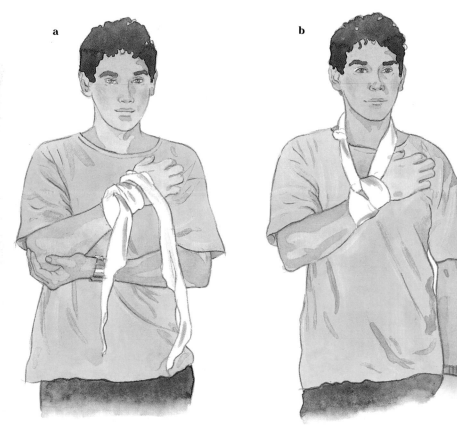

1.7 a-b Applying a collar and cuff sling

The St John sling

This supports the elbow and prevents the arm from pulling on an injured shoulder or collarbone:

☐ lay the casualty's arm naturally by the side with the elbow bent and the forearm across the chest. The fingers should point to the opposite shoulder

☐ place an open triangular bandage over the forearm and hand, with the point to the elbow and the upper end over the uninjured shoulder

☐ support the limb and tuck the base of the bandage under the fingers, hand, wrist and forearm, making a trough

a

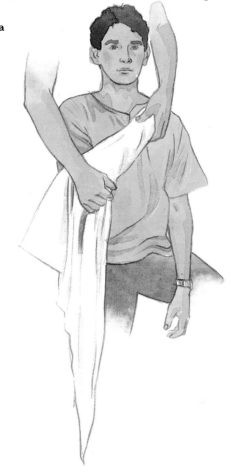

- carry the lower end around the back to the front of the uninjured shoulder. Gently adjust the height of the sling
- tie the ends as close to the fingers as possible
- tuck the point firmly in between the forearm and the bandage
- when you are sure that the sling is firm, secure the fold with a safety pin.

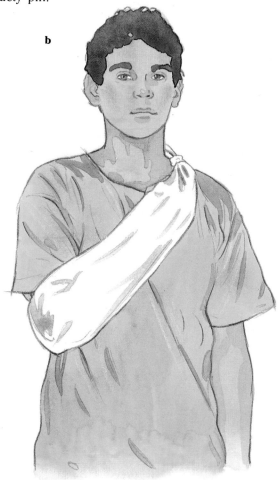

1.8 a-b Applying a St John sling

The arm sling

This is used for injuries to the forearm and wrist:

□ place an open triangular bandage over the chest with the point towards the elbow on the injured side

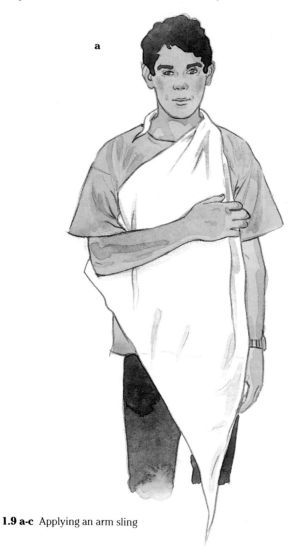

1.9 a-c Applying an arm sling

- take the upper end of the bandage over the shoulder on the uninjured side. Bring the injured arm slightly above the horizontal position
- tie the lower end to the upper end in the hollow above the collar bone on the injured side. Carefully arrange the bandage so that the fingers are showing
- fold the corner by the injured elbow and secure it with a safety pin. Check the circulation by applying gentle pressure to a finger nail. When you stop pressing it, normal colour should return rapidly to the nail bed.

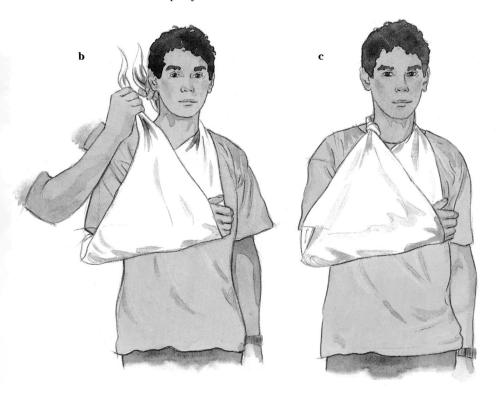

Remember: check if bandages are too tight. You may notice:
- absent pulse below the bandage
- swelling
- paleness or blueness of the fingers or toes
- numbness and tingling ('pins and needles') of the fingers or toes
- pain.

If bandages are too tight, they must be loosened. Recheck for these signs at regular intervals, or if the person complains of tightness.

2

Safety

All first aiders should be safety conscious. Safety rules and commonsense help to prevent accidents. Use these checklists to determine your level of safety awareness, and to identify changes that should be made to make your environment a safer place.

In the home

Have you:
- ☐ checked your home for objects that may cause injury?
- ☐ placed eye level markings on glass doors?
- ☐ selected safe toys for your children and ensured that they are kept in safe condition?
- ☐ stored firearms safely and out of reach of children?

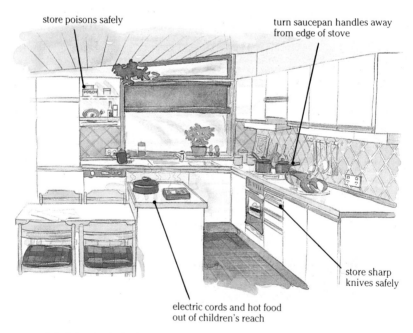

store poisons safely

turn saucepan handles away from edge of stove

store sharp knives safely

electric cords and hot food out of children's reach

2.1 Safety in the kitchen

- ☐ attached non slip backings to rugs to prevent falls?
- ☐ checked electrical goods regularly for unsafe wear?
- ☐ stored poisonous substances out of reach of children?
- ☐ destroyed unwanted medicines by returning them to your chemist or flushing down the toilet (except where there is a septic system)?
- ☐ provided your children with clothing made from non-flammable material and of a form-fitting design if likely to be near open fires or radiators?
- ☐ provided a guard for fires or radiators?
- ☐ stored plastic bags safely?

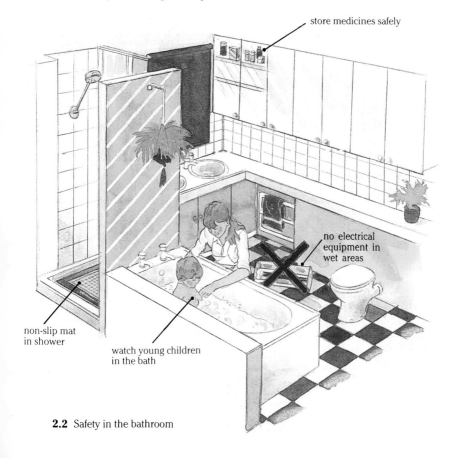

2.2 Safety in the bathroom

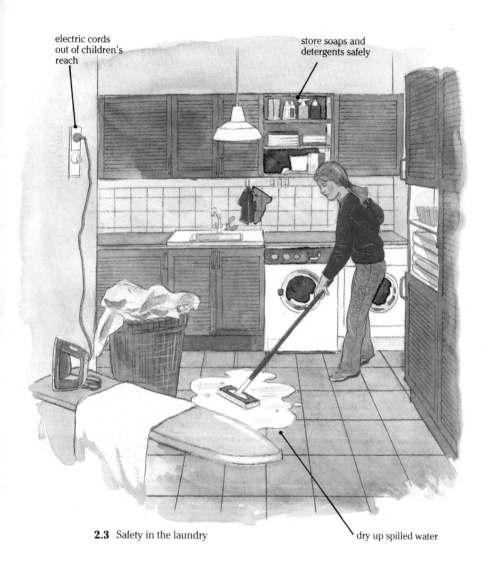

electric cords
out of children's
reach

store soaps and
detergents safely

2.3 Safety in the laundry

dry up spilled water

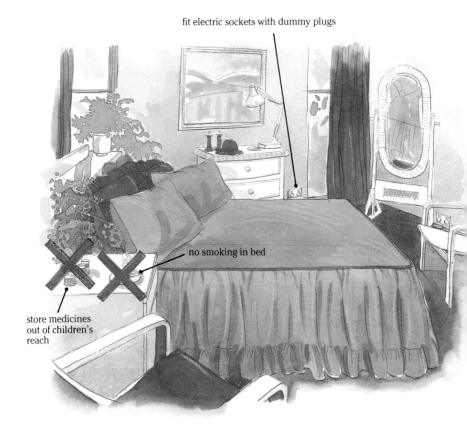

fit electric sockets with dummy plugs

no smoking in bed

store medicines
out of children's
reach

2.4 Safety in the bedroom

In case of fire

Do you:
- [ ] have the emergency telephone number handy?
- [ ] have a fire extinguisher in a central place (not near the stove)?
- [ ] have a fire blanket or woollen blanket in the kitchen for use on burning oil?

□ know the safety rules in case of fire?
  • call the fire brigade from a neighbour's home
  • if safe, shut all doors and windows
  • turn off all electric power
  • assemble all people who evacuate the building at one point
  • extinguish the fire if possible.

Outdoors

Do you:
□ regularly update first aid skills and knowledge if you have a swimming pool?
□ wrap broken glass with thick layers of paper before discarding?
□ store pool chemicals away from petroleum products?
□ label and store poisons, e.g. weedkillers, kerosene, safely?

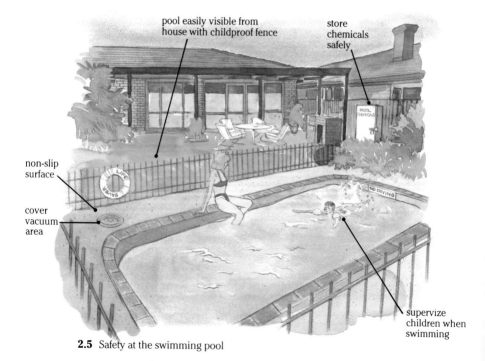

2.5 Safety at the swimming pool

- [ ] have your car, caravan and trailer checked regularly for roadworthiness?
- [ ] ensure children are in full view when reversing the car?
- [ ] ensure children are never left unattended in a car?

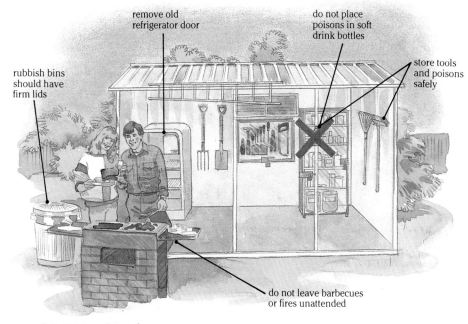

2.6 Safety in the garden

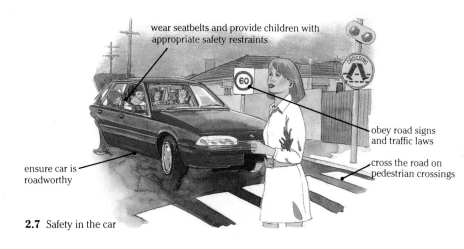

2.7 Safety in the car

Water sports

Do you:
- ☐ carry safety equipment and sufficient fuel and water when boating?
- ☐ know the distress signals and local regulations for boating?
- ☐ check the boat and ensure the engine is in good working order before use?
- ☐ ensure that there are no petrol spills or leaks when boating?
- ☐ always tell someone where you are going and what time you expect to be back when boating?

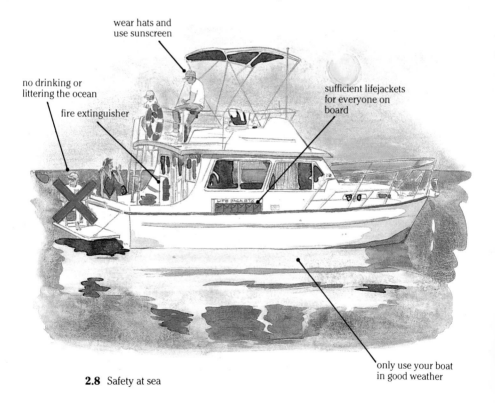

wear hats and use sunscreen

no drinking or littering the ocean

fire extinguisher

sufficient lifejackets for everyone on board

only use your boat in good weather

2.8 Safety at sea

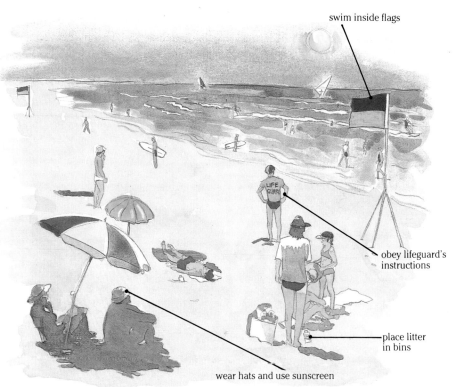

swim inside flags

obey lifeguard's instructions

place litter in bins

wear hats and use sunscreen

2.9 Safety at the beach

- ☐ consider other people, both swimming and in small boats, and always slow down near them?
- ☐ avoid swimming in isolated rivers or dams unless accompanied by other people?
- ☐ thoroughly investigate swimming holes before entering the water?
- ☐ avoid diving in unknown rivers or dams until sure of the water depth and absence of obstacles?
- ☐ ensure that you can easily get out of a swimming hole before entering?

In the bush

Do you:
- ☐ always hike or camp with companions?
- ☐ inform someone about where you are going, when you plan to arrive and return?
- ☐ take water, matches, a compass and a map of the area?
- ☐ wait for help if lost and keep together with other members of the party?
- ☐ label all dangerous items clearly and make sure that stoves and lanterns are safe?
- ☐ ensure that containers of hot food cannot be tipped over?
- ☐ ensure that collapsible tables and chairs are safe?
- ☐ wear appropriate clothes and thick-soled shoes?
- ☐ protect yourself against sunburn and insect bites?
- ☐ make sure your camp fire is out before leaving?
- ☐ know how to prevent overexposure to heat or cold?

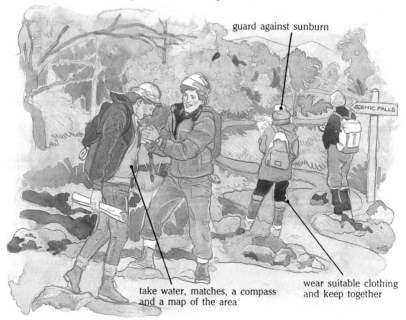

guard against sunburn

SCENIC FALLS

take water, matches, a compass and a map of the area

wear suitable clothing and keep together

2.10 Safety in the bush

In the desert

Do you:

- □ carry adequate supplies of water? At least 4 litres per person are required for drinking each day in hot weather
- □ know how to lay adequate signals for rescuers if an emergency does occur in remote desert country?
- □ know the rules for survival in the desert?
- □ take a CB radio for communication purposes?

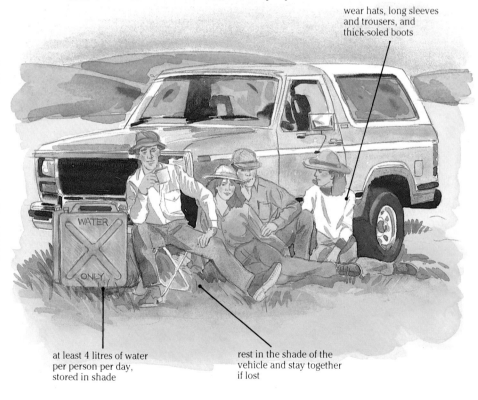

wear hats, long sleeves and trousers, and thick-soled boots

at least 4 litres of water per person per day, stored in shade

rest in the shade of the vehicle and stay together if lost

2.11 Safety in the desert

In the workplace

Are:
- ☐ working conditions safe?
- ☐ all personnel safety aware?
- ☐ safety and first aid officers trained?

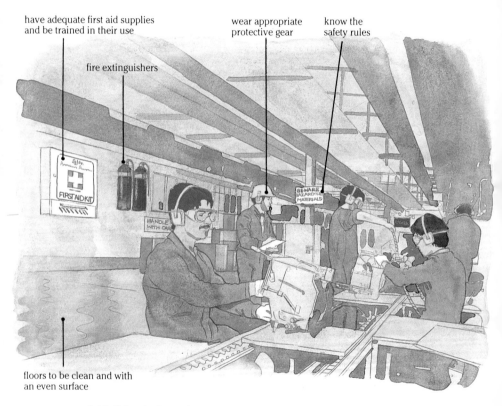

have adequate first aid supplies
and be trained in their use

wear appropriate
protective gear

know the
safety rules

fire extinguishers

floors to be clean and with
an even surface

2.12 Safety in the workplace

Everyone has a responsibility to be alert to possible dangers and to prevent accidents.

3

The DRABC
Action Plan

Danger

Response

Airway

Breathing

Circulation

When you approach the scene of an accident or emergency, follow the DRABC Action Plan:

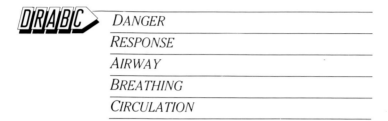

DANGER

RESPONSE

AIRWAY

BREATHING

CIRCULATION

D Check for DANGER

— to you
— to others
— to the casualty
- make sure that no one else gets hurt. You will not be able to help if you are also a casualty
- only proceed if it is safe to do so.

R Check RESPONSE

— is the casualty conscious?
- gently shake the casualty and ask: 'Can you hear me?', 'What is your name?'
- if the casualty is **conscious**, check for and manage bleeding and other injuries
- if the casualty is **unconscious**, he/she should be turned on the side.

Turning an unconscious casualty on the side to clear and open the airway

1 Kneel beside the casualty.

2 Place the casualty's farther arm at a right angle to the body.

3 Place the nearer arm across the chest.

4 Bend the nearer knee up.

5 Roll the casualty away from you. Support the casualty in this position until airway and breathing have been checked.

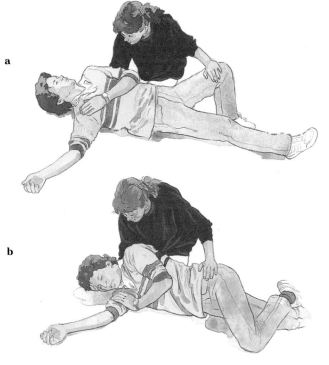

a

b

3.1 a-b Turning an unconscious casualty on the side

A *Clear and open the AIRWAY*

Clearing the airway

1 With the casualty supported on the side, tilt the head backwards and slightly down.

2 Open the mouth and clear any foreign objects. Only remove dentures if loose or broken.

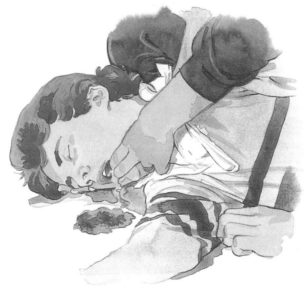

3.2 Clearing the airway

Opening the airway

1 Place one hand high on the casualty's forehead.

2 Support the chin with the other hand.

3 Gently tilt the head backwards.

4 Lift the jaw forward and open the casualty's mouth slightly.

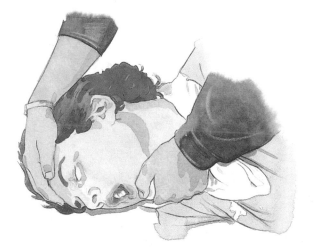

3.3 Opening the airway

B Check for BREATHING

— look for the chest rising and falling
— listen for the sound of breathing
— feel with your cheek
- if the casualty is **breathing**, ensure that he/she is in a stable side position. Check for and manage bleeding and other injuries
- if the casualty is **not breathing**, turn onto the back and commence EAR (expired air resuscitation), giving 5 full breaths in 10 seconds.

Placing an unconscious casualty in a stable side position

1 Adjust the upper knee so that the thigh is at a right angle to the hip.

2 Place the upper arm across the elbow of the lower arm.

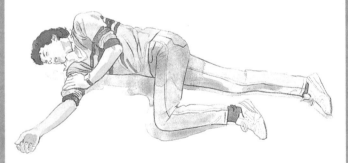

3.4 Placing an unconscious casualty in a stable side position

EAR (mouth-to-mouth resuscitation)

1 Kneel beside the casualty.

2 Keep the casualty's head tilted back.

3 Pinch the casualty's nostrils with your fingers or seal with your cheek.

4 Lift the jaw forward and upward with your other hand. Avoid pressure on the neck.

5 Take a deep breath and open your mouth wide.

6 Place your mouth firmly over the casualty's mouth making an airtight seal.

3.5 a

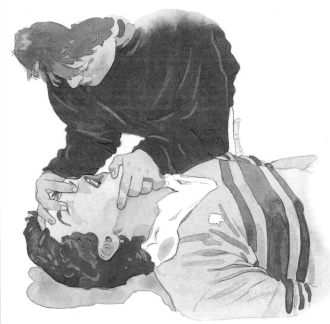

CONTINUED

CONTINUED

EAR (mouth-to-mouth resuscitation)

7 Breathe firmly into the casualty's mouth to inflate the lungs.

8 Remove your mouth and turn your head to observe the chest fall and to listen or feel for exhaled air.

9 If the chest does not rise and fall, check head tilt position first, then check again for foreign objects in the airway. If a foreign object is present, turn the casualty on the side, clear the airway, reposition, and recommence expired air resuscitation.

10 Give 5 full breaths in 10 seconds, then check the carotid (neck) pulse for 5 seconds. If pulse is present, continue EAR at the rate of 15 breaths per minute.

b

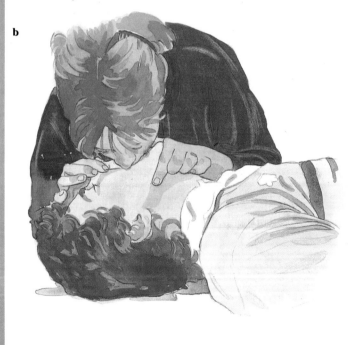

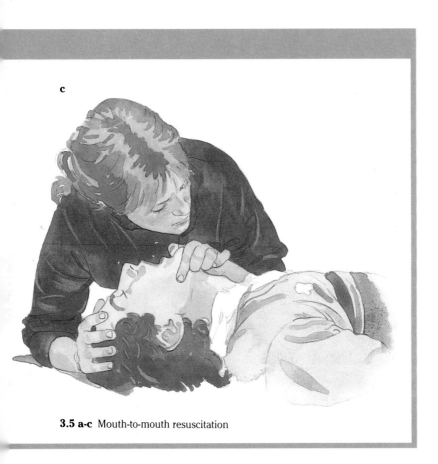

3.5 a-c Mouth-to-mouth resuscitation

C *Check for CIRCULATION*

- feel the pulse at the neck (carotid pulse)
- if pulse is present, continue EAR at the rate of 15 breaths per minute. Check breathing and the pulse after 1 minute, then after every 2 minutes
- if pulse is not present, commence CPR (cardiopulmonary resuscitation)
- check breathing and the pulse after 1 minute, then after every

2 minutes. If the pulse returns, continue EAR. If breathing returns, turn the casualty to a stable side position. Check for and manage shock, bleeding and other injuries

- seek medical aid.

To feel for the pulse

1 Place the ends of your fingers in the groove behind the Adam's apple, on either side of the neck, but not on both sides at the same time.

2 Do not use your thumb or finger tips.

3 The pulse can also be felt at the wrist (radial pulse).

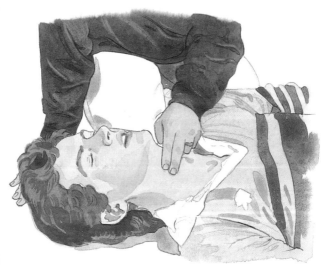

3.6 Feeling for the pulse

CPR for adults — one first aider

1 After finding that there is no pulse, kneel beside the casualty with one knee level with the casualty's chest and the other level with the head.

2 Your hands must be positioned correctly:
- locate the lower end of the breastbone by running your fingers along the lowest rib on each side from the outside inwards

3.7 a

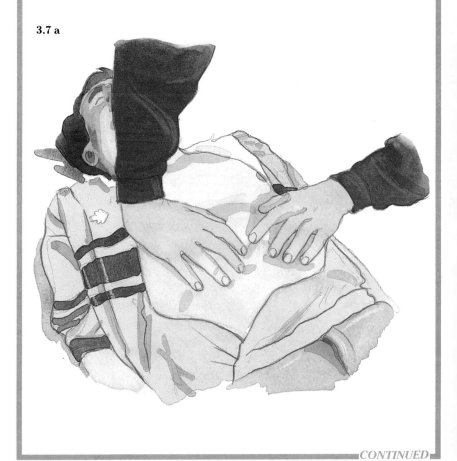

CONTINUED

CONTINUED

CPR for adults — one first aider

- locate the upper end of the breastbone by placing a finger in the groove between the collarbones
- extend the thumbs of each hand equal distances to meet in the middle
- keep the thumb of one hand in position and place the heel of the other hand below it, on the lower half of the breastbone.

b

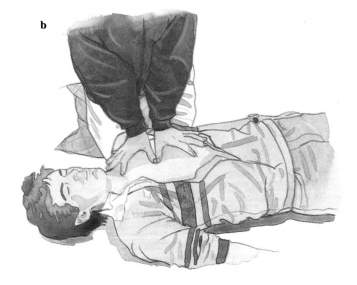

3 Your fingers should be relaxed, pointing across the chest, and slightly raised.

4 Place your other hand securely on top of the first. Lock the top thumb around the lower wrist, or interlock the fingers.

5 Exert pressure through the heel of your lower hand. Your shoulders should be above the breastbone and your compressing arm should be straight. Pivoting from the hips, perform the compressions rhythmically with equal time for compression and relaxation.

6 The breastbone should be depressed about 5 centimetres. Release the pressure.

7 Give 15 compressions in 10–12 seconds. Then give two breaths in 3–5 seconds. Continue at 4 cycles per minute.

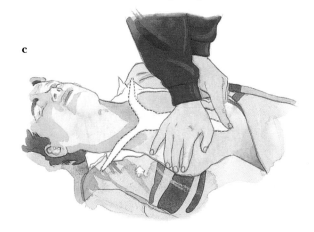

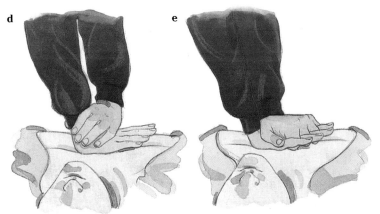

3.7 a-e Positioning the hands for CPR

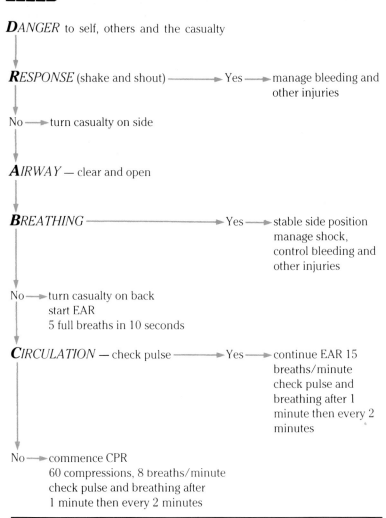

DRABC *summary*

DANGER to self, others and the casualty

RESPONSE (shake and shout) ──────► Yes ──► manage bleeding and
                                                other injuries

No ──► turn casualty on side

AIRWAY — clear and open

BREATHING ──────────────────► Yes ──► stable side position
                                          manage shock,
                                          control bleeding and
                                          other injuries

No ──► turn casualty on back
       start EAR
       5 full breaths in 10 seconds

CIRCULATION — check pulse ──────► Yes ──► continue EAR 15
                                              breaths/minute
                                              check pulse and
                                              breathing after 1
                                              minute then every 2
                                              minutes

No ──► commence CPR
       60 compressions, 8 breaths/minute
       check pulse and breathing after
       1 minute then every 2 minutes

Successful CPR

If a casualty is not breathing and has no pulse, you should try to give cardiopulmonary resuscitation. However, even if performed expertly, you may not be successful in saving the casualty's life. Success depends on the cause of the injury or illness, how quickly you are able to respond, and how quickly expert medical aid arrives. Call medical aid as soon as possible.

What next?

After managing life-threatening problems, turn the casualty to a stable side position. Remember that you must call medical aid as soon as possible. You should then undertake an orderly assessment of the casualty, looking for any bleeding, then other injuries such as burns and fractures. Note any tenderness, swelling, wounds or deformity.

Examine the casualty in the following order:
- head and neck
- chest (including shoulders)
- abdomen (including hip bone)
- upper limbs
- lower limbs
- back.

4

More about resuscitation

Expired air resuscitation

Cardiopulmonary resuscitation

An alternative method for turning
a casualty to a stable side position

EAR

Mouth-to-nose method

The mouth-to-nose method is used when:
- the jaw and/or teeth are broken
- the jaws are tightly clenched
- resuscitating in deep water
- resuscitating an infant or child when your mouth can cover the casualty's nose and mouth.

Mouth-to-nose method

1 Kneel beside the casualty.

2 Keep the casualty's head tilted back.

3 Close the casualty's mouth and place your thumb on the lower lip to keep the mouth closed. Support the jaw.

a

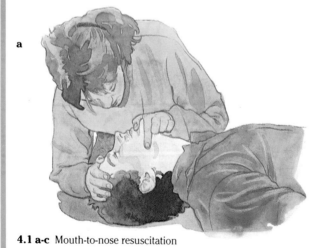

4.1 a-c Mouth-to-nose resuscitation

4 Take a deep breath and open your mouth wide.

5 Seal your mouth around the casualty's nose without compressing the soft part.

b

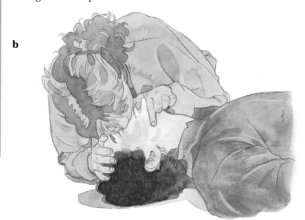

6 Breathe into the casualty's nose.

7 Remove your mouth after breathing in. Open the casualty's mouth with your thumb to allow exhalation.

c

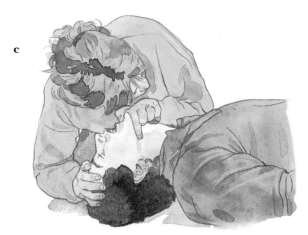

Mouth-to-mask method

The mouth-to-mask method avoids mouth-to-mouth contact between the first aider and the casualty by the use of a resuscitation mask. However, resuscitation should not be delayed by attempts to obtain a mask. An appropriate face mask is provided in the St John Ambulance Australia Communicable Diseases Protection Pack.

Mouth-to-mask method

1 Position yourself either beside the casualty's head or at the casualty's head, facing the feet. Use both hands to hold the jaw forward, maintain an open airway and to hold the mask in place.

2 Place the narrow end of the mask on the bridge of the nose. Apply the mask firmly to achieve an effective seal.

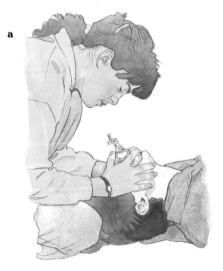

a

4.2 a-c Mouth-to-mask resuscitation

3 Take a deep breath and blow through the mouthpiece of the mask. Remove your mouth to allow exhalation. Turn your head to listen and feel for the escape of air.

4 If the chest does not rise, recheck head tilt, jaw support and mask seal.

b

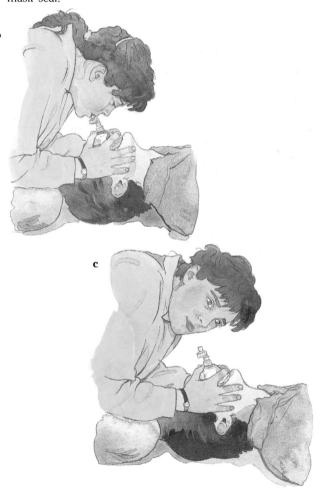

c

Babies and small children under the age of eight

After clearing the airway, support the jaw without tilting the head backwards. Do not press on the soft tissues under the chin. Cover the mouth and nose with your mouth and puff gently, using just enough pressure to make the casualty's chest rise. Too much pressure may distend the stomach. Repeat 20 times per minute.

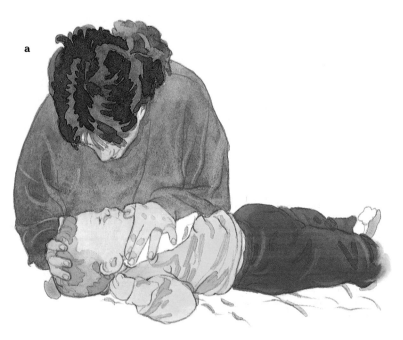

4.3 a-b EAR for babies and small children

b

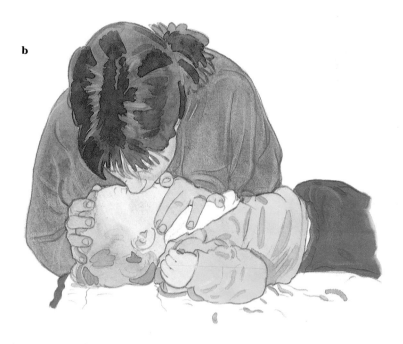

Cardiopulmonary resuscitation

CPR — two first aiders

The most experienced first aider should perform EAR. Kneeling on opposite sides of the body give 5 compressions and 1 breath in 5 seconds. Continue at 12 cycles per minute without pausing between cycles.

CPR — babies and small children under the age of eight

For a baby under the age of 1 year, use two fingers over the lower half of the breastbone, compressing to a depth of 1–2 centimetres. For a small child between the ages of 1 and 8, use the heel of one hand only, to a compression depth of 2–3 centimetres.

With one first aider, give 2 breaths to 15 compressions in 10 seconds (6 cycles per minute).

With two first aiders, give 1 breath to 5 compressions in 3 seconds (20 cycles per minute).

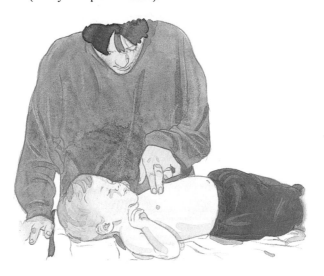

4.4 CPR for babies

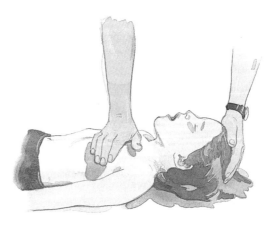

4.5 CPR for small children

An alternative method for turning a casualty to a stable side position

Kneel beside the casualty and place his nearer arm, palm up, under the buttocks. Cross the farther leg over the nearer leg and place the farther arm across the chest.

4.6 a

b

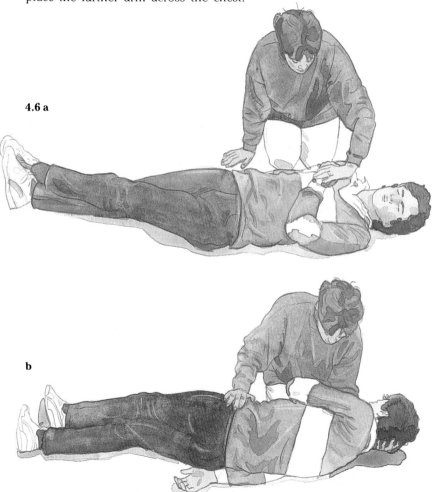

Support the casualty's head and neck with one hand. With your other hand, grasp the casualty's farther hip and roll the casualty towards you until he rests against your knees. Support the casualty in this position until airway and breathing have been checked.

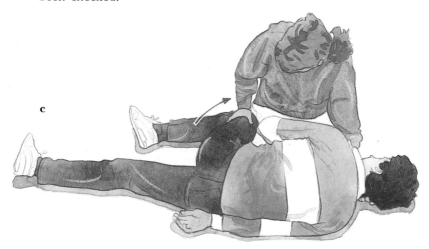

To ensure a stable side position, remove the farther arm from under the body, place the casualty's hand under the cheek, and bend the upper leg at a right angle to the body.

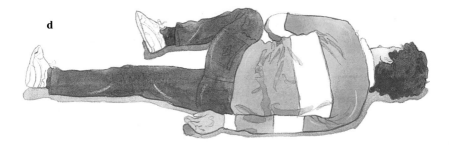

4.6 a-d Turning a casualty to a stable side position (alternative method)

5
Shock

Shock is the term used to describe a life-threatening condition that can occur as a result of serious injury or illness, particularly when there is pain, severe bleeding, or fluid loss from burns. It is a progressive condition that may lead to the collapse of the circulatory system and death. The circulatory system consists of the heart and blood vessels. Blood is circulated to all parts of the body, supplying food and oxygen, and removing waste products.

Causes

- if blood is lost, as a result of external or internal bleeding, the volume of blood in the blood vessels becomes insufficient
- fluid lost from the tissues as a result of severe burns, diarrhoea or vomiting, is replaced by fluid from the blood, thus reducing the volume of blood
- damage to the heart, e.g. as a result of heart attack
- decreased blood pressure, e.g. as a result of spinal cord injury, severe pain, infection or poisoning.

A combination of these factors may result in more severe shock.

Symptoms and signs

Immediately after injury, there may be little evidence of shock. The symptoms and signs will develop progressively, depending on:
- the severity of the injury
- continuation of fluid loss
- effectiveness of management.

Initial symptoms and signs are:
- pale face, fingernails and lips
- cold, clammy skin
- usually a weak, rapid pulse
- rapid breathing
- faintness or dizziness
- nausea.

Symptoms and signs of severe shock are:

- restlessness
- thirst
- extremities become bluish in colour
- the casualty may become drowsy, confused or unconscious
- rapid breathing
- usually an extremely weak, rapid pulse.

Management

☐ DRABC and control severe bleeding

☐ reassure the casualty

☐ seek medical aid urgently

☐ unless fractured, raise the casualty's legs above the level of the heart

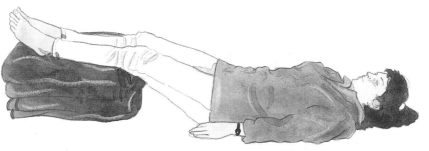

5.1 Managing shock

☐ dress any wounds or burns

☐ immobilize any fractures

☐ loosen any tight clothing

☐ keep the casualty comfortable by maintaining body warmth but do not heat

☐ if the casualty complains of thirst, moisten lips, but do not give anything to eat or drink

☐ monitor and record breathing and pulse at regular intervals. Maintain a clear and open airway

□ place casualty in a stable side position if there is breathing
   difficulty, if vomiting is likely, or if the casualty becomes
   unconscious.

6

Bleeding

Bleeding is a loss of blood from the blood vessels. Severe or continued bleeding may lead to collapse and death. Thus, the first aider must aim to control severe bleeding.

The total quantity of blood in the human body varies according to size. An adult can lose 500 ml of blood without any harm, but the loss of 300 ml might cause death in an infant.

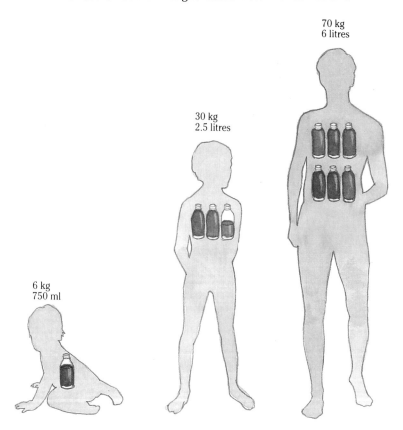

70 kg
6 litres

30 kg
2.5 litres

6 kg
750 ml

6.1 The quantity of blood in the human body

Remember: severe bleeding is serious. The extent of bleeding may be hidden. **Act quickly!**

External bleeding

Symptoms and signs

- obvious bleeding.

Management

- ☐ DRABC
- ☐ lay casualty down
- ☐ apply direct pressure to the site of bleeding
- ☐ raise and rest the injured part when possible
- ☐ loosen tight clothing
- ☐ give nothing by mouth
- ☐ seek medical aid urgently.

Direct pressure

1 Apply direct pressure to the wound with your fingers or hand.

6.2 a

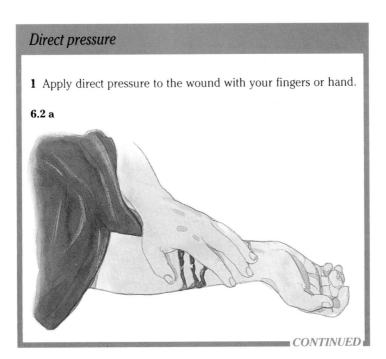

CONTINUED

CONTINUED

Direct pressure

2 As soon as possible, place a clean dressing over the wound. Apply a bulky pad extending beyond the edges of the wound, and firmly bandage. If bleeding continues, leave the dressing in place and relocate the pad.

b

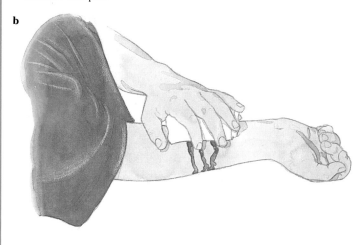

c

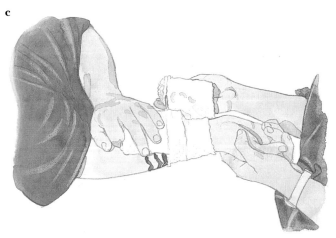

d

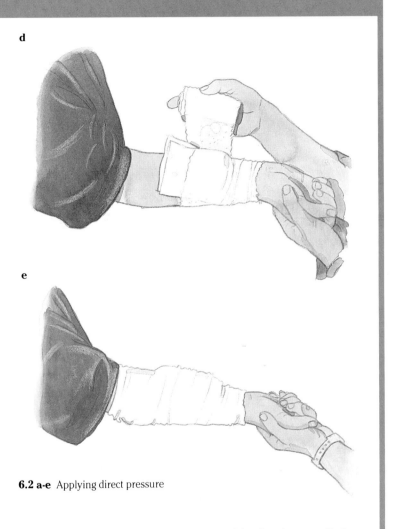

e

6.2 a-e Applying direct pressure

3 Do not disturb pads or bandages once bleeding is controlled.

Uncontrolled bleeding

If severe bleeding cannot be controlled by direct pressure, it may be necessary to apply pressure to the pressure points. These are found on the main artery above the wound. When bleeding has been controlled, remove pressure to the point and reapply direct pressure to the wound.

Occasionally, in major limb injuries such as partial amputations and shark attack, severe bleeding cannot be controlled by direct pressure. Only then, it may be necessary to resort to the application of a constrictive bandage above the elbow or knee.

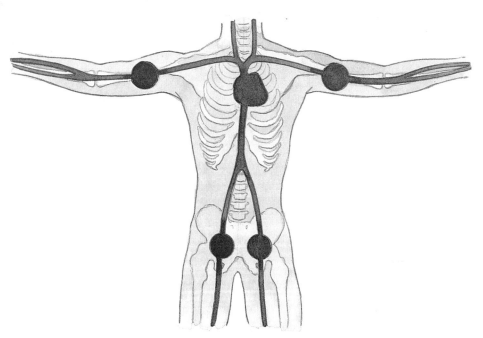

6.3 Pressure points

Using a constrictive bandage

1 Select a strip of firm cloth, at least 7.5 centimetres (3 inches) wide and about 75 centimetres (30 inches) long. This may be improvized from clothing or a narrow folded triangular bandage.

2 Bind the cloth strip firmly around the injured limb above the bleeding point until a pulse can no longer be felt beyond the constrictive bandage and bleeding is controlled. Tie firmly.

3 Note the time of application. After 30 minutes, release the bandage and check for bleeding. If there is no bleeding, remove it. If bleeding recommences, apply direct pressure. If this is unsuccessful, reapply the constrictive bandage, and recheck every 30 minutes.

4 Ensure that the bandage is clearly visible and inform medical aid of the location and time of its application.

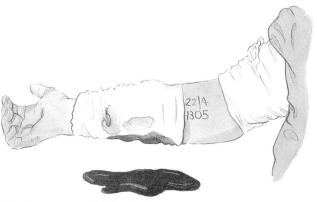

6.4   Applying a constrictive bandage

Internal bleeding

Symptoms and signs

Evidence of internal bleeding from some organs may be seen by the first aider. For example:

- coughing up red frothy blood
- vomiting blood the colour of coffee grounds or bright red. The blood may be mixed with food
- passing of faeces with a black, tarry appearance
- passing of faeces which are red in colour
- passing urine which has a red or smoky appearance.

Concealed bleeding within the abdomen may be suspected when there is:

- pain
- tenderness
- rigidity of abdominal muscles.

Internal bleeding will be accompanied by any of the following symptoms and signs:

- faintness or dizziness
- restlessness
- nausea
- thirst
- weak, rapid pulse

- cold, clammy skin
- rapid, gasping breathing
- pallor
- sweating.

Management

- ☐ lay the casualty down, or if the casualty is coughing up frothy blood, allow him/her to adopt a position of comfort (normally half sitting)
- ☐ raise the legs or bend the knees
- ☐ loosen tight clothing
- ☐ seek medical aid urgently
- ☐ give nothing by mouth
- ☐ reassure the casualty.

7

Wounds

Abrasions

Abrasions, e.g. gravel rash, occur as a result of falls on hard, rough surfaces. Dirt may be embedded in the wound and infection may follow.

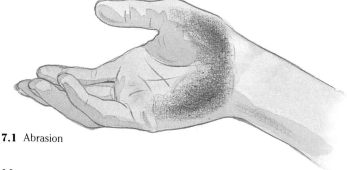

7.1 Abrasion

Management

☐ cleanse the wound thoroughly with sterile gauze soaked in sterile or cool boiled water. An antiseptic may be used according to directions on the label to help wound cleaning
☐ if this is not possible, wash the wound under running tap water
☐ gently apply a non-stick dressing.

Open wounds

Management

☐ DRABC
☐ control bleeding
☐ clean the wound as well as possible
☐ apply a sterile or clean dressing
☐ seek medical aid.

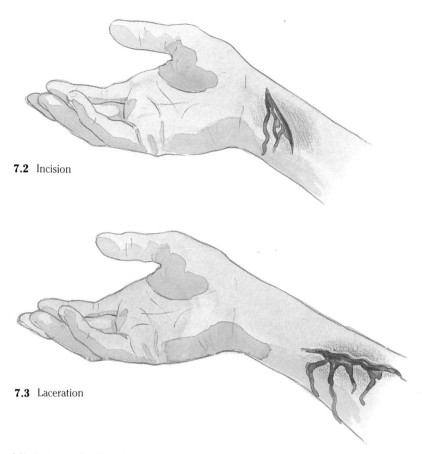

7.2 Incision

7.3 Laceration

Minimize infection by:
- washing your hands well before and after management
- avoiding coughing, sneezing or talking while managing a wound
- handling the wound only when it is necessary to control severe bleeding
- using sterile or clean dressings.

Dirty and penetrating wounds should be examined by a doctor, as tetanus or other serious and fatal infections may result.

Penetrating wounds

Penetrating wounds are serious and may occur when an object, e.g. a bullet, nail, or needle, penetrates the skin. The penetration may be deep and infection may occur.

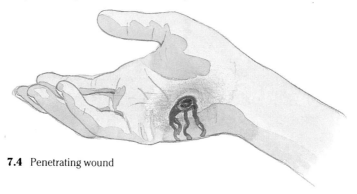

7.4 Penetrating wound

Management

☐ control bleeding by applying direct pressure around the wound
☐ keep the wound as clean as possible
☐ cut away or remove clothing covering the wound
☐ if not bleeding, carefully clean out loose dirt
☐ do not try to pick out foreign material embedded in the wound
☐ apply a sterile or clean dressing
☐ rest the injured part in a comfortable position
☐ always seek medical aid.

Crater wounds

These occur when large amounts of tissue are suddenly torn from the body. Severe bleeding and shock may result.

Management

- ☐ pack wound with sterile or clean material
- ☐ apply direct pressure and firmly bandage
- ☐ raise and rest the affected part
- ☐ seek medical aid urgently.

Foreign objects in wounds

Management

Foreign objects, e.g. gravel, lying on the surface of a wound may be lightly brushed from the wound.

If the foreign object penetrates into tissue:

- ☐ do not attempt to remove it as this may result in severe bleeding or may damage deep structures
- ☐ control bleeding by applying pressure to the surrounding areas but not on the foreign body
- ☐ place padding around the object or place a ring pad over the object and a bandage over the ring pad
- ☐ if the length of the object is such that it is protruding outside the ring pad, take care to bandage only each side of the pad
- ☐ seek medical aid.

Do not:

- exert any pressure over the object
- try to shorten the object unless its size makes it unmanageable.

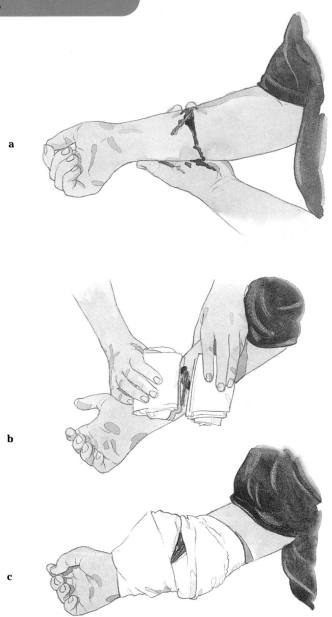

7.5 a-c Managing a foreign object in a wound

Fish hook wounds

Do not remove fish hooks, but seek medical aid.

If aid is not readily available and the hook is embedded just under the skin, attempt to remove it. Only one attempt should be made. If unsuccessful, manage as for a foreign body in the wound.

Removing a fish hook

1 Push the barb through the skin.

2 Cut off the shank of the hook and pull the hook out by the barb, or cut off the barb and pull the hook out by the shank.

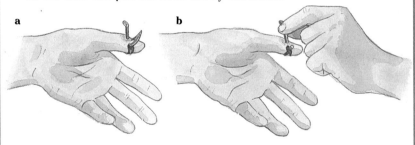

3 An alternative method is to loop a piece of fishing line around the hook and with your thumb, press the eye of the hook down. Grasp the line firmly and jerk it sharply.
Warning: the hook will fly off in the direction of the tug.

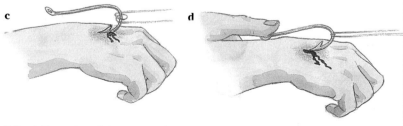

7.6 a-d Removing a fish hook

Bleeding from the palm of the hand

Bleeding may be severe as several blood vessels may be involved.

Managing bleeding from the palm of the hand

1 Immediately apply firm pressure to the palm of the hand using a pad held in place by the casualty. A firmly folded handkerchief or triangular bandage, an unopened roller bandage, a clean cloth wrapped around an object such as a matchbox, a smooth stone, or two or three fingers of the other hand may be used.

2 Elevate the hand above the head.

3 Bandage firmly over the hand and fingers with a broad roller or triangular bandage to maintain the pressure. One method of applying this bandage is to:

  □ place a bulky pad on the wound and ask the casualty to grasp it firmly

  □ place the casualty's hand on an open triangular bandage

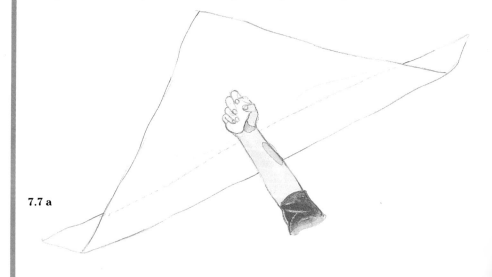

7.7 a

☐ fold the point of the triangular bandage over the clenched fist

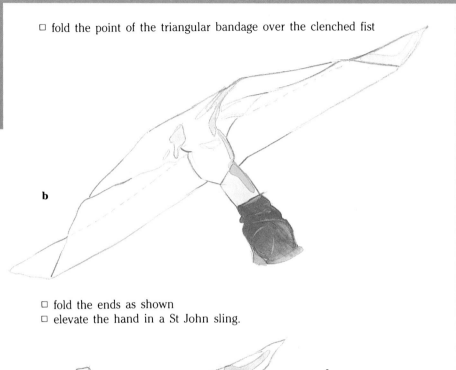

b

☐ fold the ends as shown
☐ elevate the hand in a St John sling.

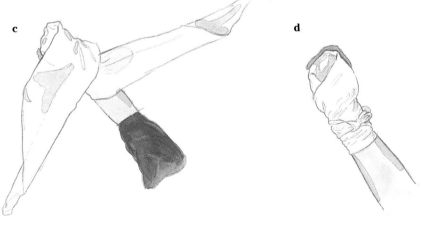

c

d

CONTINUED

CONTINUED

Managing bleeding from the palm of the hand

4 Support in a St John sling.

e

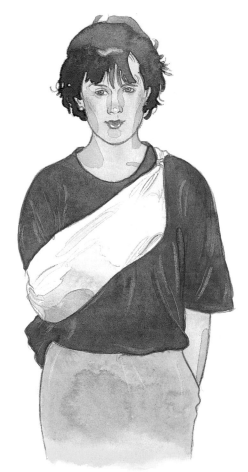

7.7 a-e Managing bleeding from the palm of the hand

Bleeding from the scalp

If the casualty's general condition and other injuries permit, sitting up may help reduce bleeding. Direct pressure may need to be maintained as it is difficult to bandage the scalp firmly enough.

Bleeding from varicose veins

Management

- □ place the casualty flat with the legs raised
- □ remove any constricting bands from the limb
- □ apply a clean pad and firmly bandage
- □ seek medical aid.

Amputated parts

Management

- □ do not wash or soak the amputated part in water or any other liquid
- □ wrap the part in gauze or material and place in a water-tight container, such as a sealed plastic bag
- □ pack the container in crushed ice added to water
- □ the part should **not** be in direct contact with ice
- □ send to hospital with the casualty.

8

Burns

Causes

Burns may be caused by:
- excessive heat, e.g. fire, steam, hot objects or liquids
- friction, e.g. rope burn
- chemicals, e.g. acids
- electricity, e.g. domestic, high voltage
- radiation, e.g. sun, microwaves, sun lamps.

Effects

Burns may result in:
- death of the superficial layers of the skin or, in severe cases, the whole skin and deeper tissues
- damage to the superficial blood vessels with outpouring of fluid, seen as blisters if the skin is intact
- a raw area, which may lead to infection
- severe pain
- the injured area becoming red, swollen and blistered
- shock.

When to seek medical aid

Extensive burns are dangerous and may be fatal. Seek medical aid if:
- the burn is deep (full thickness) — the skin may look white, or it may be black and charred. The casualty may not feel pain
- a superficial burn (a red, painful area which may blister) is larger than a 20 cent piece
- the burn involves the airway, hands, face or genitals
- you are unsure about how serious the burn is.

Rescue of the burnt casualty

Rescue can be dangerous — leave to expert help, if available.

If entering a burning building:
- feel the temperature of the door. If very hot do not enter. If cold or slightly warm, crouch low and open slowly
- cover mouth and nose with damp cloth

If domestic voltage electricity is involved:
- switch off the current or jerk the cable free
- if this is not possible, remove the casualty from the current using non-conducting, dry materials, e.g. dry clothing or a dry wooden stick
- do not cut the cable.

If high voltage electricity is involved:
- wait until the current is disconnected by the appropriate electricity authority
- ensure you and any bystanders are safe
- do not touch the casualty or any conducting material which is also in contact until the current is disconnected.

Management

- □ DRABC
- □ remove the casualty from danger. Do not become another casualty yourself
- □ put out burning clothing. Smother with a blanket or jacket, or use water
- □ hold the burnt area under cold, gently running water until the part has returned to normal body temperature (up to 10 minutes)
- □ remove jewellery and clothing, but leave any that is stuck
- □ cover the burn with a sterile, non-stick dressing
- □ seek medical aid urgently

- if the casualty is conscious and thirsty, give frequent small amounts of water. Do not give alcohol
- alleviate extreme pain by gently pouring cold water over the dressing.

a

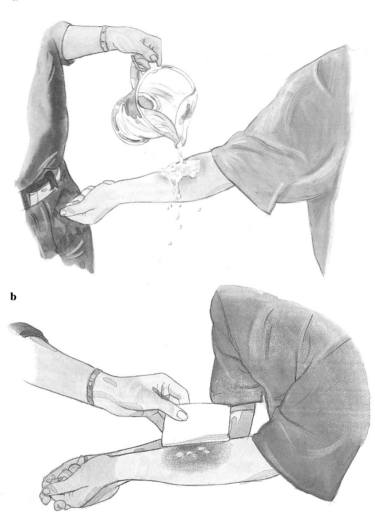

b

c

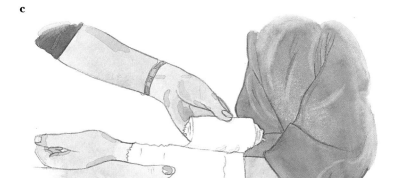

8.1 a-c Managing a burn

Warning

- **Do not** apply any lotions, ointments or oily dressings

- **Do not** prick or break blisters

- **Do not** give alcohol to drink

- **Do not** overcool the casualty, particularly if very young, or if the burnt area is extensive. Overcooling may be indicated by shivering

- **Do not** use towels, cotton wool, blankets or adhesive dressings directly on the wound.

Fires

In a fire, check for and manage:
- asphyxia (lack of oxygen) *falta*
- carbon monoxide poisoning
- poisoning from the inhalation of gases given off by plastics and synthetic building materials, e.g. PVC and polyurethane
- burns to the airway
- irritation to the respiratory tract and eyes from smoke and chemical fumes.

Sunburn *por Sol*

Take care to prevent sunburn.

Management

- ☐ cold showers
- ☐ apply cool moist compresses to the burnt area
- ☐ rest in a cool place
- ☐ cool drinks
- ☐ young babies and casualties with blisters need medical aid.

Chemical burns *químicos*

Management

- ☐ DRABC *mirar por peligro*
- ☐ wash off immediately with a large volume of flowing water for 20 minutes
- ☐ remove contaminated clothing and footwear **but avoid contaminating yourself**

- do not attempt to pick off contaminants that stick to the skin
- cover the area with a sterile or clean non-stick dressing
- seek medical aid urgently.

Electrical burns

While the surface skin may show little or no evidence of burning, deep tissues may be seriously burnt.

Management

- DRABC
- remove casualty from danger
- wash and cool burnt area under gently running water well away from live wire ~~alambee~~
- apply a sterile, non-stick dressing
- seek medical aid urgently for all electrical burns.

Bitumen burns

Management

- **do not attempt to remove bitumen from the skin or from the eyes**
- drench the burnt area immediately with cold, running, water. Use iced water if available
- apply cold wet towels frequently to maintain the cooling effect
- continue the cooling for 30 minutes, but no longer
- if the burn is to the eye, flush the eye with water for 20 minutes and cover both eyes
- seek medical aid urgently.

9

Limb injuries

Bruises

Sprains

Strains

Dislocations

Fractures

Limb injury can involve damage to bones, joints, ligaments, muscles, the major blood vessels and nerves of the limb. Depending on the severity, limb injuries may be life-threatening, or cause considerable pain and long term disability. Blood loss and shock may result, particularly in cases of multiple injury.

Bruises

These may be caused by falls, blows or crushing. Bleeding into the deep tissues occurs, causing bruising.

Symptoms and signs

- pain
- swelling
- bruising
- tenderness.

Management

☐ RICE.

RICE management

R – Rest the casualty and the injured part.

I – Ice packs wrapped in cloth may be applied to the injury — 20 minutes on and reapplied every 2 hours for the first 24 hours, then every 4 hours for a further 24 hours.

C – Compression bandages, e.g. elastic bandages, should be applied to extend well beyond the injury.

E – Elevate the injured part.

Sprains

A sprain occurs when a joint is forced beyond its normal range of movement, stretching or tearing the ligaments that hold it together.

Symptoms and signs

- pain, which may be quite intense and which will also cause restriction of movement and loss of function
- swelling
- bruising, which may develop quickly.

Management

If in doubt, manage as a fracture.

- □ DRABC
- □ RICE
- □ seek medical aid.

Strains

A strain is the result of overstretching of a muscle or tendon.

Symptoms and signs

- pain in the region, usually sharp and with sudden onset
- additional pain on movement, or if the muscle is stretched
- loss of power
- tenderness over the muscle
- sometimes a gap in the muscle.

Management

- □ DRABC
- □ apply a cold pack over the injured area
- □ advise the casualty not to further overstretch the muscle
- □ support the injured muscle with a compression bandage
- □ encourage gentle exercise to reduce painful spasm and/or shortening of the muscle
- □ avoid all rubbing or massage.

Dislocations

A dislocation occurs when force stretches the ligaments so far that the bones in the joint are pushed out of normal contact with each other.

Symptoms and signs

- pain
- inability to move the joint
- deformity
- tenderness over the joint
- rapidly developing swelling and discoloration about the joint.

Management

If in doubt, manage as a fracture.

- □ DRABC
- □ do not attempt to reduce the dislocation
- □ if a limb:
  —check the pulse and if absent, gently move the limb to try to restore circulation. Seek medical aid urgently
  —rest the joint in the most comfortable position
  —elevate if possible

—expose the joint and apply cold packs
—use soft padding and bandages to support the joint in the position in which it was found
□ for shoulder dislocations, support the shoulder and arm in the position of least discomfort and apply ice packs.

Fractures

A fracture is a broken or cracked bone. The break is usually complete, but in the young the bone can be bent without breaking completely. This is called a greenstick fracture. Correct first aid management of fractures, in both conscious and unconscious casualties, is essential, in order to reduce the amount of tissue damage, bleeding, pain and shock.

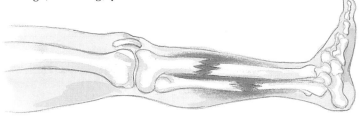

9.1 Fractured bone

Causes

- direct force — a blow that breaks the bone at the point of impact
- indirect force — when the bone breaks at some distance from the point of impact, e.g. where a fall on an outstretched hand results in a fracture of the collarbone
- abnormal muscular contraction — a sudden contraction of a muscle may result in a fracture, e.g. an elderly person snapping the kneecap after tripping and trying to prevent a fall.

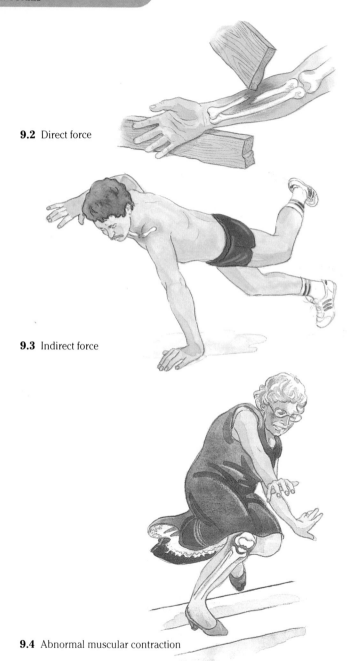

9.2 Direct force

9.3 Indirect force

9.4 Abnormal muscular contraction

Effects

- bleeding — fractures of large bones may result in considerable loss of blood, e.g. a fractured thigh results in the loss of 1 or 2 litres
- damage to surrounding tissues and blood vessels
- pain
- possibly shock.

Types

- closed — skin is unbroken and blood is lost into tissues
- open — a wound leads to the fracture, or bone protrudes through the skin. Blood loss may be severe, and infection can result
- complicated — vital organs may be damaged, e.g. rib fracture with an injury to the lung.

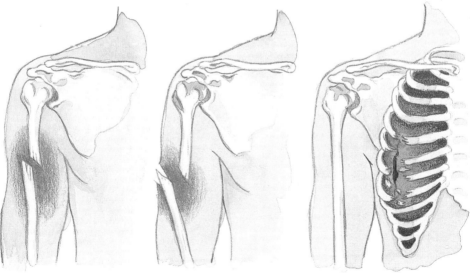

9.5 Closed fracture   **9.6** Open fracture   **9.7** Complicated fracture

Symptoms and signs

- the break may have been felt or heard
- pain at or near the site of the injury
- difficult or impossible normal movement of the limb
- loss of power
- deformity, abnormal twist or shortening of limb
- tenderness when gentle pressure is applied

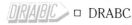

- swelling over the fracture, and possibly around it
- bruising
- a coarse grating sound if one end of the bone moves against the other. Never actively seek this sign as further injury may result.

Management — general rules

- DRABC
- control bleeding and cover all wounds
- check for fractures — open, closed or complicated
- ask the casualty not to move the injured part
- immobilize fractures with slings, bandages or splints to prevent movement at the joints above and below the fracture
- watch for signs of loss of circulation to the foot or hand
- move the casualty only if there is danger to you or the casualty
- handle gently
- observe casualty carefully and manage shock if necessary
- seek medical aid.

Methods for immobilizing a fracture

Bandages

1 Use broad bandages where possible.

2 Pass bandages under the natural hollows of the body

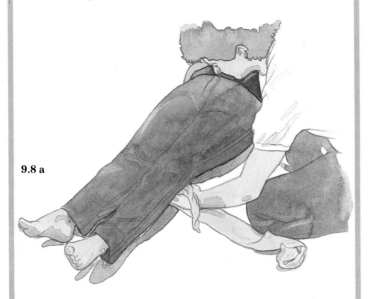

9.8 a

3 Always support the limb, applying gentle traction until bandages are secured tightly.

4 Every 15 minutes, check that bandages are not applied too tightly.

5 Check that bandages are not so loose that they will slip or fail to support the fracture.

Splints

6 A splint can be any firm material that is long enough to extend beyond the joints at either end of the broken bone.

CONTINUED

CONTINUED

Methods for immobilizing a fracture

7 Padding should be placed between the splint and the natural curves of the limb.

b

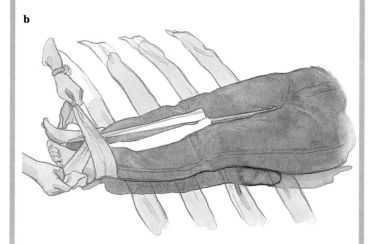

8 Place bandages at each end of the limb, and just above and below the fracture. Secure the furthest bandage first, then the bandage at the other end of the limb, followed by the bandages above and below the fracture. Non-slip knots, such as a reef knot, should be tied on the uninjured side.

c

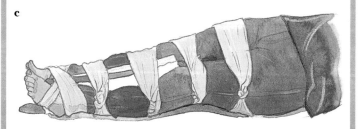

9.8 a-c Immobilizing a fracture

Fractured collar bone

Symptoms and signs

- pain, made worse by movement of the shoulder
- history of a fall onto the outstretched arm or elbow
- the casualty may support the arm at the elbow and incline the head towards the injured side
- the shoulder appears to be lower than the uninjured side
- tenderness and swelling around the collarbone.

Management

- □ DRABC
- □ follow the general rules for fracture management
- □ support the arm on the injured side in a St John sling
- □ seek medical aid.

Fractured upper arm

Symptoms and signs

- pain
- loss of function
- swelling
- the casualty may support the injured arm below the fracture.

Management

- □ DRABC
- □ follow general rules for fracture management.

If the injury is close to, or involves the elbow:
- □ lay the casualty down, supporting the injured area
- □ check the pulse at the wrist and the colour of the hand and fingers

- [ ] gently place the injured limb on supporting material by the side of the body. Do not bend the elbow
- [ ] immobilize the arm firmly to the body with broad bandages
- [ ] tie bandages in front on the uninjured side
- [ ] check the pulse
- [ ] seek medical aid.

a

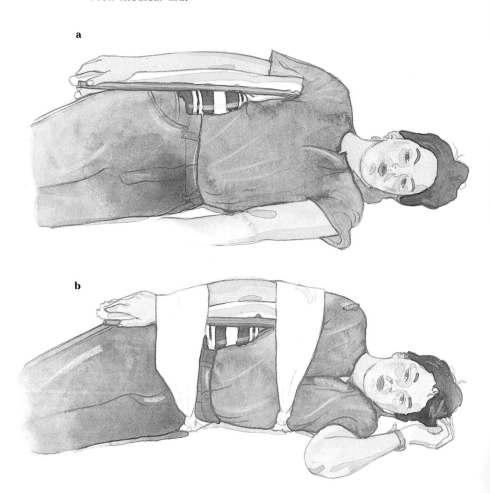

b

9.9 a-b Managing a fractured upper arm (close to elbow)

If the injury is not close to the elbow:

☐ apply a collar and cuff sling

☐ do not support under the elbow. Allow the elbow to hang freely

☐ place soft padding between the elbow area and the chest

☐ immobilize the arm with two broad bandages (or narrow ones for a small person):

—one above the fracture, over the arm and around the chest

—the other below the fracture

☐ tie off the bandages in front on the uninjured side

☐ check the pulse

☐ seek medical aid.

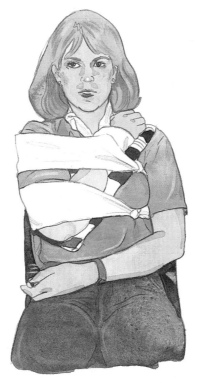

9.10 Managing a fractured upper arm (not close to elbow)

Fractured forearm

Symptoms and signs

- pain
- loss of power
- deformity
- the casualty may support the injured forearm with the other arm.

Management

- □ DRABC
- □ follow the general rules for fracture management.

If the fracture is **not** near the elbow:
- □ immobilize the limb firmly to a splint which extends from the elbow to the fingers. Bandage:
  —above the fracture, below the elbow
  —below the fracture
  —at the wrist/hand
- □ apply an arm sling
- □ seek medical aid
- □ check pulse and colour of fingers.

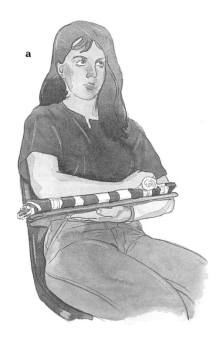

a

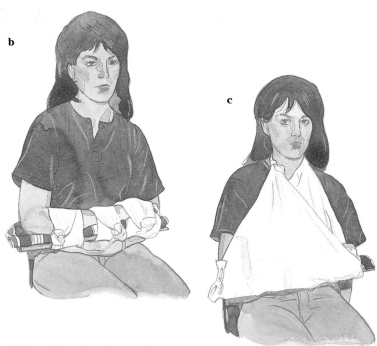

9.11 a-c Managing a fractured forearm

If the fracture is near the elbow:
- □ immobilize the arm in the position found
- □ check the pulse
- □ seek medical aid urgently.

Fractures of the hands and fingers

Symptoms and signs

- pain
- swelling
- deformity
- bleeding, if there is a wound.

Management

Hand fractures

- ☐ DRABC
- ☐ place soft padding between the chest and the limb
- ☐ apply a St John sling
- ☐ support the arm with a broad bandage over the forearm, tied off on the uninjured side
- ☐ check pulse
- ☐ seek medical aid.

Finger or thumb fractures

- ☐ DRABC
- ☐ rest the injured hand on a well padded splint and secure with a bandage
- ☐ elevate the hand for as long as possible
- ☐ during transport, support the hand in a St John sling
- ☐ seek medical aid.

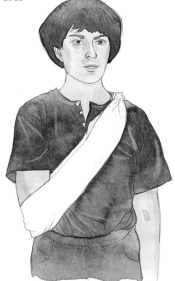

9.12 Managing a fractured finger or thumb

Fractured wrist

Symptoms and signs

- usually a history of a fall on an outstretched hand
- pain and swelling
- tenderness
- weakness of the hands and fingers
- deformity often present.

Management

☐ children may prefer to support their own wrist. Allow them to do so

☐ rest the forearm and hand on a well padded splint. Additional padding under the hand and wrist may be required

☐ secure the limb to the splint by bandaging below the elbow, across the back of the hand and around the middle of the forearm

☐ elevate the limb

☐ apply a large arm sling

☐ seek medical aid.

Fractured thigh

Symptoms and signs

- severe pain at the site of the injury
- loss of power
- tenderness at the site of the injury
- deformity
- swelling
- possibly a rotation of the foot of the injured leg
- possible shortening of the injured leg
- shock.

Management

 □ DRABC

□ cover open wounds

□ place padding between legs

□ gently bring uninjured limb to the injured limb

□ apply a figure-of-eight bandage around the ankles and feet

□ apply a broad bandage around the knees and tie on the uninjured side

□ seek medical aid.

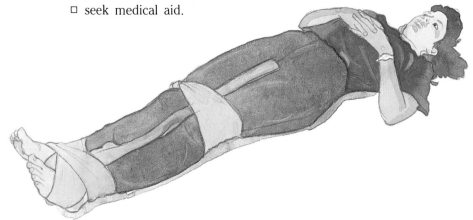

9.13 Managing a fractured thigh

If expert assistance is likely to be delayed:

 □ DRABC

□ cover open wounds

□ gently bring uninjured limb to the normal position

□ place a well padded splint between the legs

□ place one hand under the heel and the other around the toes of the injured limb

□ gently draw down to apply traction to the foot, while rotating the leg to a position as nearly normal as possible against the splint

a

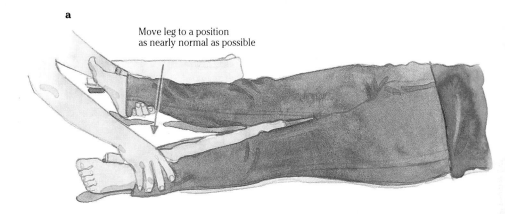

Move leg to a position
as nearly normal as possible

- apply a narrow figure-of-eight bandage around the ankles and feet
- pass bandages under:
  —the thighs above the fracture
  —the thighs below the fracture
  —both knees
  —between the knees and the ankles
- tie on the uninjured side
- check the circulation of both limbs (note the colour and temperature of the skin and feet).

b

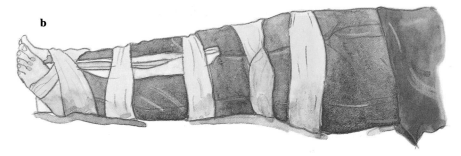

9.14 a-b Managing a fractured thigh if expert assistance is delayed

Fractured neck of the thigh bone

Symptoms and signs

- pain in the area of the hip, thigh or knee, and when moving the limb
- loss of power
- tenderness over the hip
- outward rotation of the foot of the injured leg
- shortening of the injured leg
- bruising (seen later).

Management

- DRABC
- if the casualty has been lying on the ground for a long period of time, manage any scalds to the skin from urine and faeces
- reassure the casualty
- make casualty comfortable
- place padding between legs and under tender spots
- apply a figure-of-eight bandage at the ankles and a broad bandage at the knees
- seek medical aid.

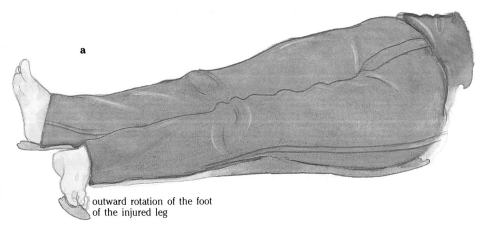

a

outward rotation of the foot of the injured leg

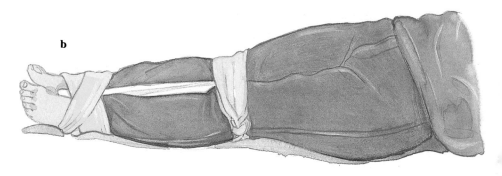

b

9.15 a-b Managing a fractured neck of the thigh bone

Fractured kneecap

Symptoms and signs

- pain over the kneecap, aggravated by movement
- loss of power at the knee
- inability to straighten the leg
- tenderness and swelling over the kneecap
- sometimes a gap can be felt at the front of the knee
- sometimes the displaced kneecap can be felt.

Management

- ☐ DRABC
- ☐ lay the casualty on the back with head and shoulders raised
- ☐ raise the leg about 30 centimetres and support it in the most comfortable position
- ☐ do not attempt to straighten the knee
- ☐ if the limb can be splinted without increasing discomfort, then
  — apply a pressure bandage around the knee (figure-of-eight crepe or conforming bandage)
  — apply a splint along the back of the limb from buttock to beyond the heel

—ensure that the splint is adequately padded, particularly under the natural hollows of the knee and ankle
—secure the limb to the splint by a figure-of-eight bandage around the ankle and foot, broad bandage around the thigh, and broad bandage around the lower leg
□ support and elevate the leg
□ seek medical aid.

a

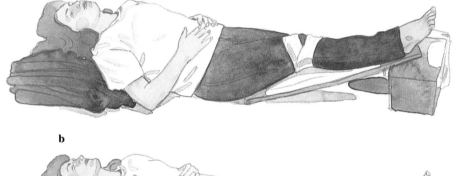

b

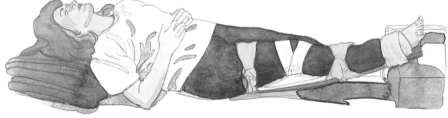

9.16 a-b Managing a fractured kneecap

Fractured lower leg

Symptoms and signs

- pain
- inability to walk
- shortening of injured leg
- deformity

- swelling
- rotation of foot of injured leg
- protruding bone
- bleeding.

Management

- DRABC
- control bleeding and cover wounds
- place padding between the legs
- bring the uninjured limb to the injured limb
- steady and support the injured limb
- apply a figure-of-eight bandage around the ankles and feet
- apply a broad bandage around the knees, and tie on the uninjured side.

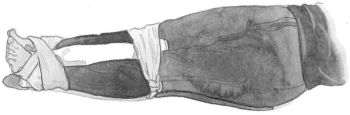

9.17 Managing a fractured lower leg

If expert assistance is delayed:

- DRABC
- control bleeding and cover wounds
- place a well padded splint between the legs, from the thighs to the ankles
- pad between the thighs, knees and ankles
- apply a figure-of-eight bandage around the ankles and feet
- apply a broad bandage around the thighs, at the knees, above and below the fracture
- seek medical aid.

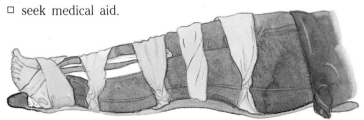

9.18 Managing a fractured lower leg if expert assistance is delayed

Fractured feet and toes

Symptoms and signs

- pain
- inability to walk
- tenderness
- swelling.

Management

- □ DRABC
- □ only remove shoes and socks if there is an open wound
- □ if casualty is not wearing shoes, apply a compression bandage
- □ raise foot and rest on pillow
- □ seek medical aid.

Fractured ankle

This fracture may be mistaken for a sprain, particularly if no deformity is present.

Symptoms and signs

- history of a twisting injury
- pain and swelling on either or both sides of the ankle
- inability to bear weight on the ankle
- tenderness, particularly over the bony prominences on either side of the ankle
- deformity, which may be severe.

Management

If no deformity is present:
- □ RICE
- □ avoid any weight bearing on the affected limb
- □ seek medical aid.

If deformity is present:
- steady and support the injured limb on pillows or a folded blanket
- do not apply any compression bandages around the ankle
- seek medical aid urgently.

10

Head, neck and spinal injuries

Head injuries

Spinal injuries

Head injuries

Head injuries involve damage to the brain or the structures of the skull surrounding the brain. No head injury should be disregarded or treated lightly. Every casualty who has had even a mild head injury must be observed thoroughly to detect any complications. The casualty who has been unconscious for even a moment must always be advised to seek medical aid.

Special precautions

A casualty who, having recovered consciousness, lapses again into an unconscious state, is in serious and immediate danger. All casualties who are unconscious as a result of a head injury must be presumed to have suffered a spinal injury.

Causes

These include:
- car and motor cycle accidents
- a blow to the head
- a fall in which the head is struck
- landing heavily on the feet
- diving into shallow water
- contact sports.

Prevention

Wear protective head gear when:
- working on a building site
- horse riding
- motor cycle riding
- playing cricket
- cycling
- playing rugby football.

Symptoms and signs

In assessing someone for damage to the brain or a fracture to the skull, look for the following symptoms and signs:

- history of injury
- loss of memory (particularly of the event)
- headache
- blurred vision
- altered or abnormal responses to commands and touch
- wounds to the scalp or to the face
- blood or clear fluid escaping from the nose or ears
- pupils becoming unequal in size.

Management

□ DRABC

□ manage as if unconscious
  —turn to a stable side position
  —clear and open airway
  —monitor breathing and circulation
□ remember the possibility of a spinal injury: support the head and neck during movement
□ if the face is badly injured, keep the airway open with your fingers. Do not force the jaw open if clenched
□ control bleeding but **do not apply direct pressure** to the skull if you suspect a fracture
□ if blood or fluid comes from the ear, secure a sterile dressing **lightly** in place. If possible lay the casualty on the injured side
□ if there is an eye injury lightly cover both eyes with a sterile pad
□ seek medical aid urgently.

Concussion

Concussion is an altered state of consciousness, often only brief, following a blow to the head.

Symptoms and signs

- history of injury
- loss of consciousness (unable to recall events).

Management

☐ as for head injury.

Compression

This occurs when blood escaping from a broken blood vessel accumulates and compresses part of the brain.

Symptoms and signs

- deteriorating level of consciousness
- noisy and/or rapid breathing
- convulsions
- unequal and unreactive pupils
- weakness on one side.

Management

☐ as for head injury
☐ seek medical aid urgently.

Fractured base of the skull

Symptoms and signs

- bleeding or clear fluid from one or both ears
- blood in the white of the eye.

Management

☐ as for head injury
☐ support the head and neck when turning the casualty on the

side, preferably injured side down
- □ do not try to close the casualty's mouth
- □ seek medical aid.

Spinal injuries

Spinal injuries should always be regarded as serious and requiring careful management. If the casualty is not correctly handled, paralysis can result.

If you are the first person at the scene of an accident, careful assessment and management of the casualty will play an important part in minimizing permanent disability and hence, in increasing the casualty's recovery potential.

The spinal column consists of 33 bones (vertebrae) which support the body. Discs separating the vertebrae allow movement and act as shock absorbers. The vertebral column encloses a canal which houses the spinal cord, an extension of the brain. It is a complex bundle of nerve cells and fibres transmitting messages for movement and sensation to and from the brain.

If the cord is damaged, communication between the brain and the body below the injury fails, causing loss of power and sensation. Lesser injury may result in partial paralysis or altered sensation. This is usually permanent because spinal nerve cells do not recover. Death may result if vital groups of cells controlling breathing and circulation are damaged.

Displaced or ruptured discs, or bone fragments that pinch the spinal cord, may cause temporary damage.

Twisting, compressing or bending an injured spinal column may:
- worsen damage caused by the injury
- damage the cord, even if it was not damaged initially.

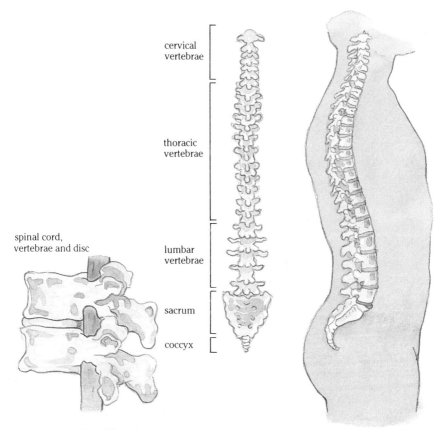

cervical
vertebrae

thoracic
vertebrae

spinal cord,
vertebrae and disc

lumbar
vertebrae

sacrum

coccyx

10.1 The spine

Causes

- motor vehicle and motor cycle accidents
- diving and watersport activities
- sporting accidents
- industrial accidents
- gunshot and knife wounds
- falls
- heavy blows to the back
- landing heavily on buttocks.

Prevention

- wear a seatbelt when driving
- wear a helmet on motor-cycles, bicycles, skateboards and construction sites
- check the water depth before diving or waterskiing
- play by the rules in sport.

Symptoms and signs

- pain at or below the site of the injury
- absent or altered sensation, e.g. tingling in the hands or feet
- loss of movement or impaired movement below the site of the injury
- tenderness over the injury site

If the casualty is unconscious as a result of a head injury, suspect a spinal injury.

Management

If the casualty is unconscious and/or suspected of having a spinal injury:

- ☐ DRABC
- ☐ maintain a clear and open airway
- ☐ if possible, before turning the casualty on the side, apply a cervical or improvized collar to minimize movement of the neck in any direction.

If the casualty is conscious:

- ☐ reassure
- ☐ loosen tight clothing
- ☐ do **not** move the casualty unless essential because of danger
- ☐ unless circumstances make it necessary, leave lifting, loading and transportation to a qualified person, such as an ambulance officer
- ☐ support the head and neck by placing your hands on either side of the casualty's head until other support can be

arranged. This is especially important if the casualty is found in a sitting position, as when trapped in a motor car
☐ apply a cervical collar if available, or improvize by using a folded towel, newspaper or other bulky dressing around the neck
☐ seek medical aid urgently.

a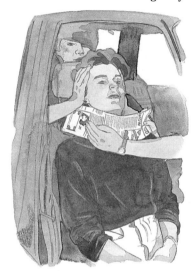

b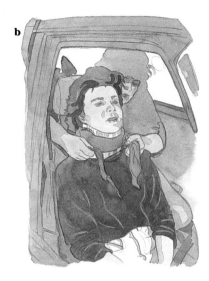

c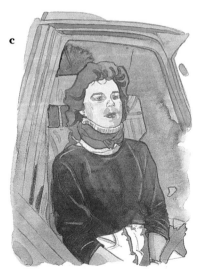

10.2 a-c Managing a conscious casualty with a spinal injury

When a diving accident has occurred:

- □ use a flotation aid or surf board, if handy, to support the casualty before removing from the water
- □ leave the casualty on the board until medical aid arrives.

Cervical collars

1 Apply a cervical collar to minimize movement of the neck in any direction

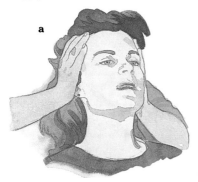
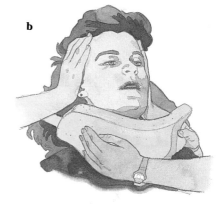

10.3 a-b Applying a cervical collar

2 Applying an improvized cervical collar — a folded towel, newspaper or other bulky dressing can be used.

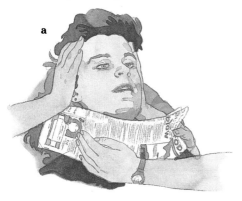
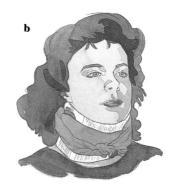

10.4 a-b Improvizing a cervical collar

11

Facial injuries

Facial injuries can potentially result in severe disability, including the loss of the senses of sight, hearing or smell. The first
aider must aim to protect the eyes, ears and nose of all
casualties, particularly the unconscious.

The eye

The eye is very susceptible to infection. Always wash your hands
carefully before managing a casualty with an eye injury. Most
eye injury management requires both eyes to be covered.
Remember that this may cause the casualty to become
disoriented.

Foreign objects in the eye

These may include:
- loose eyelashes
- insects
- grit or dust
- glass
- cosmetics
- metal particles.

Symptoms and signs

- pain in the eye, particularly when looking at light
- gritty feeling in the eye
- watering of the eye
- redness of the eye
- inability to open the eye
- spasm or twitching of the eyelid.

Warning:
- the casualty should avoid rubbing the eye
- never try to remove a foreign object from the coloured part of the eye
- never try to remove any object that is embedded in the eye
- do not persist in examining the eye if the injury is severe.

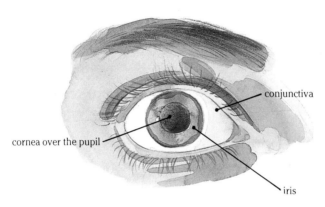

cornea over the pupil

conjunctiva

iris

11.1 The eye

Management

If a foreign object is embedded in the eye:
☐ if available, lay the casualty on a stretcher
☐ cover both eyes, ensuring that the pad does not press on the injured eye, by placing thick pads on the bony part of the eye socket above and below the eye. See illustrations overleaf.

If the foreign object is small and loose:
☐ it may be washed out by tears
☐ if not, try to remove the object as described **overleaf**.
☐ if unsuccessful, refer to medical aid.

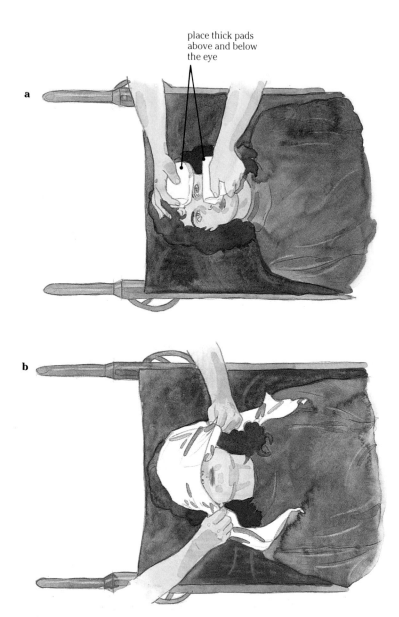

11.2 a-b Managing a foreign object embedded in the eye

Removing a small, loose foreign object from the eye

1 Ask the casualty to look up. Gently draw the lower lid down and out. If the foreign object is visible, remove it, using the corner of a clean cloth, moistened in water.

2 If the foreign object is not visible, ask the casualty to look down. Gently grasp the lashes of the upper lid. Pull the lid down and over the lower lid. This may dislodge the foreign object.

3 If the latter method is unsuccessful, wash the eye with a gentle stream of clean water or sterile saline.

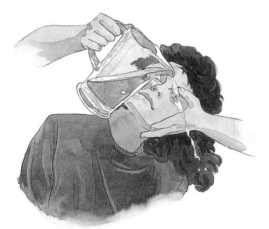

11.3   Removing a small loose foreign object from the eye

Burns to the eye

Causes

- chemicals, e.g. acids, caustic soda, lime
- heat, e.g. flames or radiant heat
- welding flash or ultraviolet light.

Symptoms and signs

- pain
- intolerance of light
- severe watering of the eyes
- reddening of the eyeball
- swollen eyelids
- in the case of welding flash, a gritty feeling and pain, which may not be felt until several hours after exposure.

Warning: in the case of chemical burns, immediate action is necessary.

Management

If a chemical or heat burn:

- ☐ DRABC
- ☐ open the eyelids gently with your fingers
- ☐ wash the eye with cold flowing water for at least 20 minutes, ensuring that you wash under the eyelids
- ☐ place eye pads or light clean dressings over both eyes
- ☐ seek medical aid promptly.

If a welding flash or ultraviolet light burn:
- ☐ place eye pads or light clean dressings over both eyes
- ☐ seek medical aid.

Smoke in the eyes

Symptoms and signs

- pain
- watering
- reddening
- the casualty may close the eyes tightly.

Management

☐ DRABC
☐ ask the casualty not to rub the eyes
☐ wash the eyes with cold tap water or sterile saline if available. The remainder of the solution will need to be discarded after use.

Wounds to the eyes

Causes

- direct blows
- fast moving objects, e.g. a squash ball.

Warning: do not persist in examining the eye if the injury is severe.

Management

☐ reassure the casualty
☐ lay the casualty on the back
☐ place a light dressing over both eyes, ensuring there is no pressure on the injured eye
☐ ask the casualty not to move the eyes
☐ arrange immediate ambulance transport to medical aid.

Contact lenses

If the casualty is wearing contact lenses and they can be easily removed, ask him to remove them before the eye injury is managed. Do not remove them yourself.

The ear

Bleeding from the ear

This may indicate a fractured base of the skull or other serious injury.

Causes

- a blow to the head
- a fall.

Management

- ☐ DRABC
- ☐ **do not** plug the ear canal
- ☐ **do not** administer drops of any kind
- ☐ allow fluid to drain freely
- ☐ place the casualty on the side with the affected ear downwards, even if the casualty is conscious
- ☐ place a sterile pad between the ear and the ground
- ☐ seek medical aid urgently.

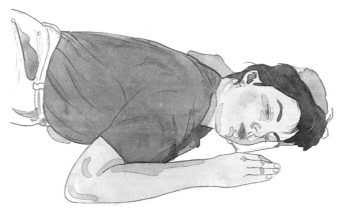

11.4 Managing bleeding from the ear

Ruptured ear drum

The ear drum is a fine membrane stretched across the channel between the outer and middle ears. It is an essential link in the chain that transmits sound to the brain. If the ear drum is ruptured the casualty has diminished hearing in that ear.

Causes

- explosions
- SCUBA diving
- pressure changes when flying
- a blow to the ear
- a foreign object in the ear
- infection.

Symptoms and signs

- pain, usually severe
- absent or diminished hearing through the affected ear
- blood or fluid escaping from the ear.

Management

- ☐ reassure the casualty
- ☐ manage as for bleeding from the ears
- ☐ seek medical aid.

Foreign objects in the ear

Small objects can become lodged in the ear, e.g.
- pins
- matchsticks
- beads
- small insects
- grass seeds.

Warning:
- do not probe the ear, but gently inspect the ear to identify the object and how deeply it is placed
- do not attempt to remove, unless a small insect.

Management
□ seek medical aid.

If a small insect:
□ place one droplet of vegetable oil, warmed to body temperature, in the ear. If vegetable oil is not available, use a little warm water
□ if the insect does not float out, seek medical aid.

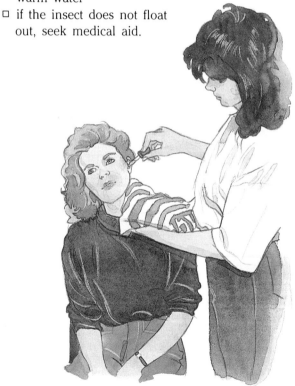

11.5 Removing a small insect from the ear

The nose

Foreign objects in the nose

These may include:

- peas
- beads
- marbles
- cotton
- seeds
- crayons.

Management

- ☐ if a small object, block the opposite nostril and ask the casualty to blow it out of the nose
- ☐ tell the casualty to breathe through the mouth
- ☐ seek medical aid.

Bleeding from the nose

Causes

- a blow to the nose
- excessive blowing of the nose.

Management

- ☐ ask the casualty **not** to blow the nose, and to breathe through the mouth
- ☐ sit the casualty up with the head slightly forward
- ☐ have the casualty apply finger and thumb pressure on the soft part of the nostrils for at least 10 minutes
- ☐ loosen all tight clothing around the neck, chest and waist
- ☐ keep the casualty cool with a supply of fresh air
- ☐ place cold wet towels on the neck and forehead
- ☐ if bleeding continues, reapply finger and thumb pressure for 10 minutes. If bleeding persists, seek medical aid.

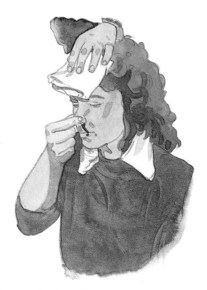

11.6 Managing bleeding from the nose

Broken nose

Symptoms and signs

- history of injury
- pain
- swelling
- bruising
- bleeding from the nostril.

Management

- ☐ seek medical aid urgently
- ☐ if bleeding, manage as for bleeding from the nose. There is no requirement for pressure unless bleeding is severe.

The jaw

Fractured jaw

Symptoms and signs

- pain
- inability to chew
- tenderness
- swelling
- deformity
- misalignment of jaw and teeth
- drooling of saliva.

Management

- □ DRABC
- □ if unconscious, turn on the side. If conscious, and other injuries permit, allow the casualty to sit in the position of greatest comfort (usually sitting up and leaning forward)
- □ support the jaw with your hand, or pull the lower jaw forward to keep the airway clear and open. The casualty may be able to support his/her own jaw if conscious
- □ seek medical aid.

Dislocated jaw

Symptoms and signs

- inability to close the mouth
- pain in front of the ear
- tenderness
- drooling of saliva.

Management

- ☐ DRABC
- ☐ remove any dentures
- ☐ support the lower jaw
- ☐ seek medical aid.

The teeth

Bleeding from a tooth socket

This may follow:
- a tooth extraction
- a blow to the mouth, in which a tooth is dislodged.

Management

- ☐ instruct the casualty to keep the tongue clear of the socket
- ☐ do not attempt to remove the clot in the socket by rinsing
- ☐ place a firm pad of gauze over the socket and instruct the casualty to bite firmly onto it
- ☐ if the bleeding continues, seek medical or dental aid.

Tooth injuries

Management

If a tooth is knocked out:
- ☐ save the tooth
- ☐ clean the tooth, by having the casualty suck it or by washing in saliva or milk. Do not handle the root of the tooth
- ☐ if possible, replace the tooth in the mouth in its original position

- □ hold in place for 2 minutes, then mould a piece of aluminium foil or milk bottle cap over it and two neighbouring teeth on each side. This acts as a temporary splint
- □ have the casualty bite firmly onto this splint for added stability
- □ if it is not possible to replace the tooth, store it in saliva or milk until dental attention is available
- □ if the tooth has been in contact with soil or dirt advise the casualty to have an anti-tetanus injection if not currently immunized
- □ advise the casualty to see a dentist as soon as possible.

If a tooth is loosened:
- □ straighten the tooth
- □ splint with foil as described above
- □ advise the casualty to see a dentist as soon as possible.

12

Chest injuries

Chest injuries range from a simple bruising of the chest with slight pain or discomfort on breathing, to life-threatening injury to the vital organs, and can seriously affect breathing and circulation.

Types of injury

- fractured ribs
- flail chest
- bruising of the lung
- penetrating chest wound
- lung injury, e.g. bleeding, collapse of the lung, leaking of air and/or blood in the chest space.

Causes

- blows, e.g. steering wheel impact
- falls
- crushing by heavy objects
- stabbing
- gunshots
- blasts.

Fractured ribs

The fracture may be closed, or ribs may be forced into, and damage the lungs. As a result, blood and air may collect in the chest space.

Symptoms and signs

- pain, worsening as the casualty breathes and coughs
- breathing difficulty. The casualty may support the injured side of the chest with his arm or hand

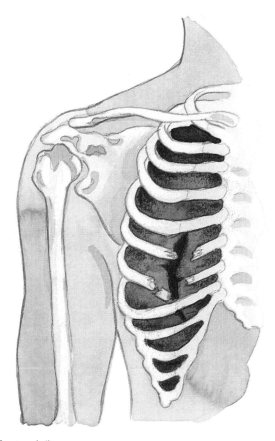

12.1 Fractured rib

- breathing may be short, rapid and gasping
- tenderness at the site of the injury
- frothy, bloodstained sputum.

escape sangre con burbujas

Management

If the casualty is conscious:

□ place the casualty in a comfortable position, normally half sitting and leaning to the injured side, if other injuries permit

- ☐ encourage the casualty to breathe with short breaths using the diaphragm
- ☐ gently place ample padding over the injured area
- ☐ apply one or two broad bandages according to the size of the casualty, securing the arm and padding to the chest on the injured side
- ☐ tie off in front on the uninjured side
- ☐ if bandages increase discomfort, loosen or remove them
- ☐ immobilize the arm using a St John sling or collar and cuff sling
- ☐ seek medical aid urgently.

If the casualty is unconscious:

- ☐ DRABC
- ☐ lay the casualty on the injured side
- ☐ seek medical aid urgently.

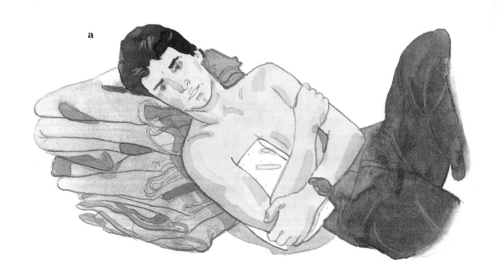

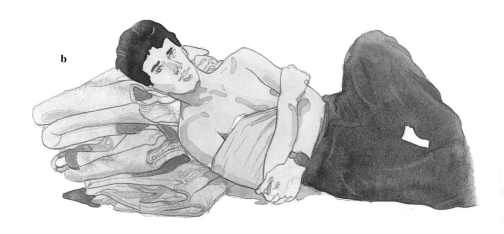

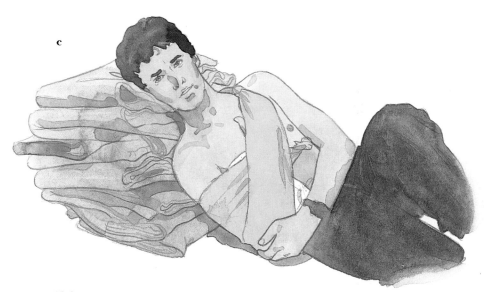

12.2 a-c Managing a fractured rib

Flail chest

This occurs when several ribs are broken in more than one place, in such a way that part of the rib cage becomes loose.

The loose part does not move with the rest of the rib cage when the casualty breathes. Instead it moves in the opposite direction. This is called **paradoxical breathing**.

Symptoms and signs

- shortness of breath (gasping for air)
- chest pain
- breathing difficulty
- blue lips
- difficulty in speaking
- loose part moving in a direction opposite to that of normal breathing
- unconsciousness.

Management

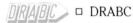

- □ DRABC
- □ clear and open airway
- □ if the casualty is conscious, place in a comfortable position, normally half-sitting, leaning to the injured side. If unconscious, turn to the injured side
- □ loosen tight clothing
- □ place a large bulky dressing over the loose area with a firm bandage
- □ bend the arm on the injured side at the elbow and with fingers pointing to the opposite shoulder, securely bandage to the chest
- □ seek medical aid urgently.

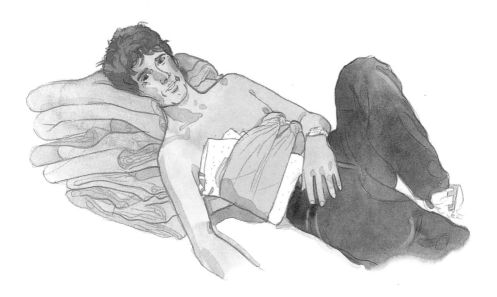

12.3 Managing a flail chest

Penetrating chest wound

This may result in air being sucked into and out of the chest cavity. The lung may collapse and blood may accumulate between it and the chest wall.

Symptoms and signs

- pain at the site of the injury
- breathing difficulty (shortness of breath)
- a wound, or blood on clothing
- sucking noise in the wound
- unconsciousness.

Management

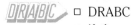

- □ DRABC
- □ if the casualty is conscious, place in a comfortable position, normally half-sitting, leaning to the injured side. If unconscious, turn to the injured side
- □ place your hand over the wound until an airtight dressing, e.g. plastic sheet, plastic bag or aluminium foil, is available
- □ tape the top and both sides of the dressing in place. **Do not** tape the bottom edge
- □ if an airtight dressing and adhesive tape are not available, cover the wound with a clean or sterile dressing. Remove it if breathing becomes more difficult
- □ seek medical aid.

13

Abdominal and pelvic injuries

Injuries of the abdomen

Injuries of the pelvis

Injury to the abdomen requires prompt medical attention. If the spleen, liver or pancreas are injured, profuse internal bleeding may result. Injury to the bowel may result in the spilling of contents into the abdominal cavity, causing inflammation. Shock is often a complication of abdominal and pelvic injuries.

Causes

- motor vehicle accidents
- sports injuries
- blunt objects
- crushing by a heavy weight
- sharp instruments
- heavy falls
- swallowed foreign bodies.

Injuries of the abdomen

Symptoms and signs

- pain
- nausea and/or vomiting
- pallor
- grunting breathing
- evidence of the injury, e.g. bruising, wound tenderness
- resistance of abdominal muscles to light pressure
- blood in the urine if the bladder is injured
- blood escaping from the anus or genitals if these have been involved
- protrusion of intestines through a penetrating abdominal wound
- development of shock.

Management

- DRABC
- loosen clothing
- place the casualty on the back with the head and shoulders slightly raised and with a blanket placed under the knees

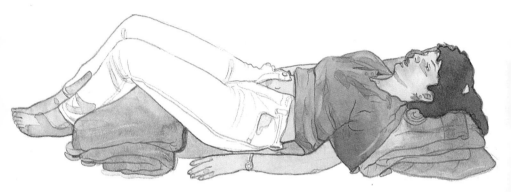

13.1 Managing an abdominal injury

- give nothing to eat or drink. If the casualty is thirsty, moisten the lips
- cover protruding intestines with a large non-stick sterile dressing, aluminium foil or plastic food wrap, preferably soaked in sterile saline, or clean water if this is not available
- seek medical aid urgently.

Swallowed foreign object

Management

- give nothing to eat or drink
- seek medical aid.

Emergencies of the abdomen

Many diseases of the abdominal organs need emergency management, e.g. appendicitis.

Symptoms and signs

- pain in the abdomen or lower back
- nausea and/or vomiting
- tenderness in the abdomen
- rapid breathing and pulse
- rigidity of abdominal muscles
- possibly, high temperature
- possibly, swelling of the abdomen
- shock.

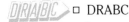

Management

- DRABC
- loosen clothing
- position the casualty as for an abdominal injury
- give nothing to eat or drink, but if the casualty is thirsty, moisten the lips
- seek medical aid urgently.

Injuries of the pelvis

Causes

- motor vehicle accidents, and in particular, those involving pedestrians
- crush injury
- fracture of the pelvis, resulting in injuries to the organs located in the pelvic area.

Symptoms and signs

- pain in the region of the hips or groin, increasing with movement
- inability to stand
- tenderness
- bruising in the groin or scrotum
- shock.

Management

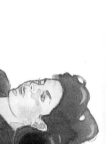

- □ DRABC
- □ if conscious, place the casualty flat on the back with the knees slightly bent and supported by a folded blanket

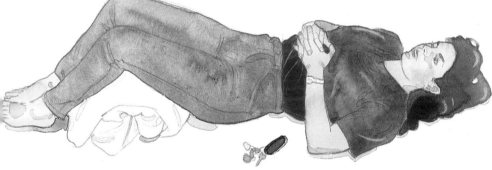

13.2 Managing a pelvic injury

- □ immobilize on a stretcher or firm support
- □ remove the pocket contents
- □ instruct the casualty not to pass urine (there may be a strong desire to do so)
- □ seek medical aid urgently
- □ reassure the casualty.

If medical aid will be delayed, or you need to move the casualty

1 Place soft padding between the knees, legs and ankles.

2 Apply a narrow figure of eight bandage around feet and ankles.

3 Apply a broad bandage around the knees.

4 Support the pelvis on either side with rolled up blankets.

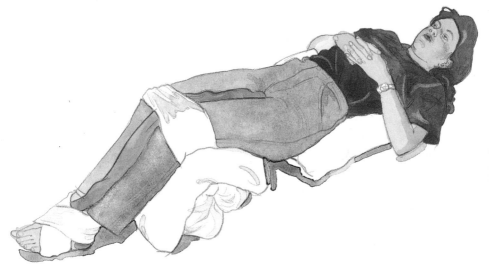

13.3 Managing a pelvic injury if medical aid is delayed

Emergencies of the pelvic organs

Causes

- retention of urine
- emergencies of the female reproductive organs
- injury of the male reproductive organs.

Retention of urine

Symptoms and signs

- pain in front of the pelvis
- extreme desire to pass urine
- swelling in the lower abdomen.

Management

- ☐ lay the casualty on the back with legs raised and a blanket or pillow under the knees
- ☐ seek medical aid urgently.

Emergencies of the female reproductive organs

Symptoms and signs

- resistance of abdominal muscles to light pressure
- pain in the lower abdomen and groin
- bleeding from the vagina
- tenderness in the lower abdomen
- shock.

Management

- ☐ lay the casualty on the back with legs raised
- ☐ seek medical aid urgently.

Injury of the male reproductive organs

Symptoms and signs

- pain
- nausea and/or vomiting
- 'doubling up' with guarding of the injured area
- swelling

- bruising *morado irritado*
- tenderness.

Management

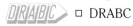 □ DRABC
□ rest and reassure casualty
□ lay the casualty on the back with knees slightly bent and supported by a folded blanket, or in a position of comfort
□ cooling of the injured area with wet cloths or ice packs may minimize bruising
□ seek medical aid.

14

Care of the acutely ill

Disorders of breathing

Asthma

Asthma is a breathing problem resulting from sudden or progressive narrowing of the airways. Attacks can be caused by:
- exercise
- allergies, e.g. pollens
- cold air
- some drinks
- preservatives
- respiratory infections
- anxiety or emotional stress
- house dust
- food additives
- stress
- smoke.

Symptoms and signs
- casualty may be sitting up
- moderate to severe breathing difficulty
- sometimes wheezing
- sometimes coughing
- possibly paleness, sweating, blueness of lips, ear lobes and fingertips
- may be very quiet or subdued
- possibly unconsciousness.

Management
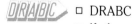
- ☐ DRABC
- ☐ if the casualty is conscious, assist him/her into the most comfortable position, usually sitting upright

- reassure the casualty
- provide assistance in administering any medications that have been prescribed for the casualty's asthma attacks
- ensure adequate fresh air
- seek medical aid
- if the casualty is unconscious, follow the DRABC Action Plan and seek medical aid urgently.

Choking

Choking is common to all age groups and is preventable.

Causes

- laughing or crying while eating or drinking
- running and stumbling while eating or drinking
- inadequate chewing of food
- swallowing splinters of bone
- inhaling while eating or drinking.

Symptoms and signs

- coughing
- violent attempts to breathe
- clutching the throat
- increasing blueness of the face, neck, lips, ears and finger-nails
- sometimes unconsciousness and absent breathing.

Management

If the casualty is conscious:
- encourage him/her to relax and breathe deeply
- ask the casualty to cough to remove the object
- if breathing is laboured, seek urgent medical aid.

If the casualty is breathing and unconscious:

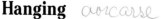

- ☐ follow the DRABC Action Plan
- ☐ seek urgent medical aid.

If the casualty is not breathing:
- ☐ lay the casualty with the head low
- ☐ give 3 or 4 sharp blows between the shoulder blades
- ☐ follow the DRABC Action Plan
- ☐ seek medical aid urgently.

Hanging

Management

- ☐ grasp the casualty's legs and take the weight of the body
- ☐ free the neck by loosening or cutting the noose
- ☐ DRABC
- ☐ seek medical aid.

Near drowning

Prevention

- learn to swim
- know safety rules for boating and swimming pools
- know basic life saving, rescue and resuscitation techniques.

Symptoms and signs

- no breathing
- blue face and lips
- possibly a fine foamy froth from the mouth and nose
- possibly no pulse.

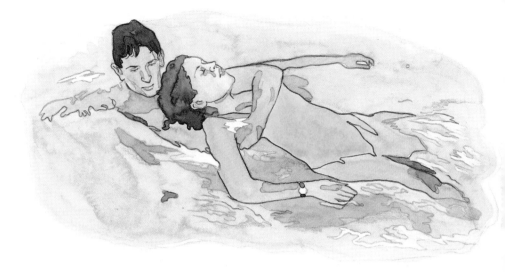

14.1   Rescuing a near-drowning casualty

Management

Warning: never attempt a rescue beyond your swimming ability. Do not become a casualty yourself.

Remember: every second is vital!

- ☐ DRABC
- ☐ check the airway and clear water, vomitus and any foreign objects if necessary
- ☐ begin mouth-to-nose resuscitation in the water (if possible) and while wading ashore. If you are in deep water, you will need a flotation aid. Do not begin EAR if your safety is jeopardized
- ☐ once ashore, check the airway again
- ☐ resume EAR
- ☐ check the pulse. If absent, begin CPR
- ☐ seek medical aid urgently

❑ if the casualty starts to breathe, and is unconscious, place on the side, keep warm and regularly observe and record pulse and breathing until medical aid arrives.

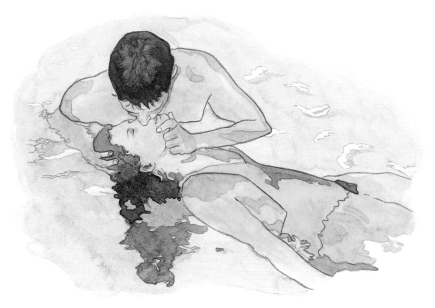

14.2 Mouth-to-nose resuscitation in water

Overbreathing

Causes

- excitement, hysteria or other emotion.

Symptoms and signs

- normal or pink skin colour
- feeling of choking, suffocation and a need to breathe deeply
- anxiety
- pins and needles in hands, feet and face
- hands may be bent at wrist with fingers straight and thumb against the fingers.

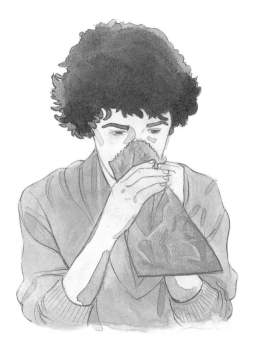

14.3 Management of overbreathing

Management

- firm reassurance *dark seguridad*
- encourage casualty to take slow, regular breaths
- instruct the casualty to breathe in and out of a paper bag until symptoms disappear.

Strangulation

Management

- remove any material constricting the throat
- DRABC
- seek medical aid.

Swollen throat tissues

Causes

- injury
- allergy
- infection
- stings and bites
- burns
- inhalation of hot gases.

Symptoms and signs

- swelling in the neck
- breathing difficulty.

Management

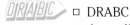 □ DRABC
□ depending on the cause, remove from smoke or allergic atmosphere

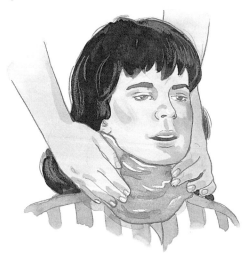

14.4 Managing a casualty with swollen throat tissues

- if the casualty is carrying any medication for this condition, e.g. for a known allergy, it should be given at once
- manage any bite or sting
- sit the casualty upright
- loosen tight clothing
- ensure plenty of fresh air
- apply ice packs to the throat
- if breathing ceases, give EAR
- seek medical aid urgently.

Disorders of consciousness

Convulsions (infantile)

Convulsions may occur in infants and young children between the ages of 10 months and 4 years. They are often associated with high body temperature resulting from a cold or other illness.

Symptoms and signs

- stiff, rigid body
- twitching limbs
- possible arching of the head and back
- rolling of the eyes
- congestion of the face and neck
- blue face and lips
- unconsciousness.

Management

- ensure a clear and open airway — if necessary turn child head down

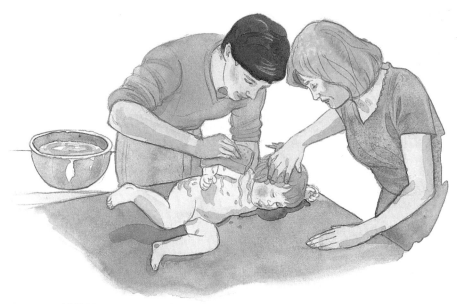

14.5 Managing a convulsion

□ remove all clothing
□ if the child feels hot, sponge down with water that is slightly below body temperature (test with your elbow)
□ fan the wet child with a newspaper or magazine to speed up cooling. Do not overcool
□ when the child has ceased convulsing and the body temperature has been reduced, cover lightly
□ reassure the parents
□ seek medical aid.

Diabetes

Diabetes is a condition caused by a disorder of the pancreas, where the body's blood sugar level becomes too high. Diabetics need a medically controlled diet and may require regular insulin

medication. Many diabetics wear or carry a medical alert brace-
let, or medical warning card. They may also have glucose or
sugar in a pocket or bag.

The first aider may encounter two types of emergencies affect-
ing diabetics — either a very low blood sugar (hypoglycaemia)
or a very high blood sugar (hyperglycaemia). Usually the emergency will occur because of very low blood sugar.

Low blood sugar

Causes

- injection of too much insulin
- not enough food containing sugar in a person who takes
  insulin
- unaccustomed exercise
- a missed meal.

Symptoms and signs

- dizziness
- weakness, trembling or shaking
- hunger
- numbness around lips and fingers
- paleness
- profuse sweating
- rapid pulse
- mental confusion (often aggressive behaviour), which, if the
  condition is untreated, may progress to unconsciousness.

Management

If the casualty is unconscious:
- □ DRABC
- □ **give nothing by mouth**
- □ seek medical aid urgently.

If the casualty is conscious:

- give sugar, glucose or a drink liberally sweetened with sugar, e.g. soft drink or cordial (not diabetic-type cordials). Continue giving sugar every 15 minutes until medical aid arrives or the casualty recovers
- loosen tight clothing
- seek medical aid.

High blood sugar

Causes

- infection in a known diabetic
- insufficient insulin.

Symptoms and signs

- excessive thirst
- frequent need to urinate
- hot dry skin
- rapid pulse
- smell of acetone on the breath (like nail polish remover)
- drowsiness
- unconsciousness.

Management

If the casualty is unconscious:

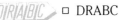

- DRABC
- seek medical aid urgently.

If the casualty is conscious:

- allow the casualty to self-administer insulin. Do not administer it for the casualty
- seek medical aid. If aid will be delayed, encourage the casualty to drink sugar-free fluids.

Epileptic seizures

Symptoms and signs

- a 'cry' as air is forced out through the vocal cords
- casualty falls to the ground, sometimes resulting in injury, and lies rigid for some seconds with back arched and jaws clenched
- congested, blue face and neck
- jerking, spasmodic muscle movement and colour improvement as breathing starts again
- froth, sometimes bloodstained, from the mouth
- casualty may bite tongue
- possibly, loss of bladder and bowel control
- casualty regains consciousness but may be confused for several minutes, and may be unaware of what happened
- after the seizure, the casualty may be exhausted and sleep deeply.

Management

- ☐ DRABC
- ☐ protect the casualty from injury, but do not restrict movement. Do not attempt to place anything in the casualty's mouth
- ☐ place the casualty on the side as soon as possible
- ☐ manage any injuries resulting from the seizure
- ☐ if the casualty falls asleep, do not disturb, but continue to check ABC
- ☐ seek medical aid. If you know that the casualty is an epileptic, seek medical aid only if the seizure continues for more than 10 minutes.

Stroke *derrame cerebral*

Symptoms and signs

- loss of movement and feeling, usually on one side of the body
- severe headache
- difficulty in swallowing
- altered level of consciousness
- slurred or garbled speech
- flushed face
- sometimes seizures
- pounding pulse
- pupils may be different size
- possibly head and eyes turned to one side
- weakness.

Management

- DRABC
- seek medical aid urgently
- reassure the casualty. He/she may be able to understand you, even if unable to communicate
- if casualty is conscious, support the head and shoulders on pillows, loosen tight clothing, maintain body temperature and wipe away secretions from the mouth. Ensure the airway is clear and open.

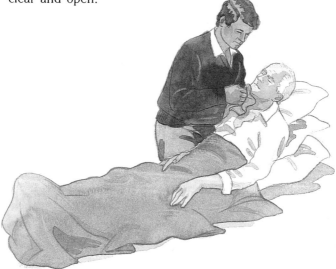

14.6 Managing a conscious casualty who has suffered a stroke

Disorders of the heart and circulation

Angina

Angina is due to narrowing of the coronary arteries. Those who suffer from angina are usually under medical treatment, and are likely to understand their problem and carry medication for use during attacks.

Symptoms and signs

- pain or discomfort in the centre of the chest which may radiate up the neck and down either arm, although commonly the left. The onset of the pain is with exercise or emotional stress and is relieved by rest or medication.

Management

- support the casualty in a sitting position
- encourage total rest and provide reassurance
- loosen tight clothing around the neck, chest and waist
- if the casualty carries tablets for angina, tell him/her to place the prescribed dose under the tongue or inside the cheek as indicated on the bottle
- if the pain or discomfort persists for longer than 10 minutes after rest it may indicate a heart attack
- angina sufferers do not normally need to go to hospital or see a doctor after an attack, provided they respond within 10 minutes to rest and/or medication. However, any adult who develops chest pain or shortness of breath should see a doctor.

Fainting

Causes

- standing still for a long time, e.g. in a hot stuffy room, or on parade
- sudden change of position, e.g. standing up after sitting
- injury (often minor)
- an unpleasant sight.

Symptoms and signs

- giddiness
- blurred vision
- weakness
- 'hot and cold' feeling
- yawning
- temporary loss of consciousness
- slow, weak pulse
- pale, cold, clammy skin.

Management

☐ lay the casualty down with legs raised, and head and body flat
☐ loosen tight clothing
☐ check for injury or illness

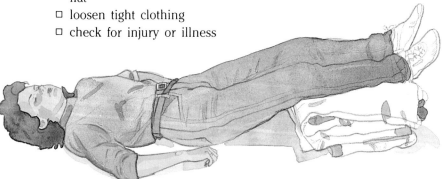

14.7   Managing a casualty who has fainted

- after recovery, let the casualty rest for some minutes before moving
- if the casualty does not recover quickly, follow the DRABC Action Plan and seek medical aid.

Heart attack

Symptoms and signs

- pain or discomfort in the centre of the chest. Pain is sometimes severe and vice-like, and radiates to the arm, or the neck and jaw. It may be confused with the pain associated with indigestion
- anxiety, confusion or distress
- nausea and/or vomiting
- shortness of breath
- pale, cold, clammy skin
- sometimes an irregular pulse
- shock may develop
- sometimes immediate collapse, leading to absence of pulse.

Management

- DRABC
- if conscious, sit the casualty up
- if pulse is weak and rapid or the person is light-headed, place casualty on the side, unless he/she is more comfortable sitting up
- if unconscious, turn the casualty on the side
- seek medical aid urgently.

Heart failure

Symptoms and signs

- acute shortness of breath
- noisy, gurgly breathing
- sometimes, chest pain
- sometimes, frothy bloodstained sputum
- rapid, weak pulse
- swollen, congested neck veins
- swollen legs and ankles
- blue lips and extremities.

Management

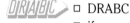

- ☐ DRABC
- ☐ if conscious, sit the casualty up
- ☐ loosen tight clothing
- ☐ reassure casualty
- ☐ seek medical aid urgently.

Sudden death

Symptoms and signs

- rapid loss of consciousness
- no breathing
- no pulse.

Management

- ☐ DRABC
- ☐ seek urgent medical aid.

15

Poisoning

General information

Poisons Information Centres

A poison is any substance that, when taken into the body, may be harmful to the normal functions of the body.

Poisons may enter the body by:
- the mouth (swallowed)
- the lungs (inhaled
- the skin (absorbed or injected).

Poisons may be solid, liquid or gaseous. They may be found in food, medications, household substances and industrial products.

Prevention

- when attempting to help a casualty, do not become a casualty yourself
- do not leave poisons or medicines within reach of children. Keep in a locked cupboard
- destroy unwanted medicines and poisons
- use properly labelled, childproof containers for medicines and poisons
- never put poisons or medications into drink bottles
- beware of poisonous fumes or gases in enclosed spaces.

Effects

The effects of poisons vary according to the substance and the amount and may be immediate or delayed.

Poisons that act most rapidly are usually those that are injected or inhaled. Those which are absorbed through the skin usually act most slowly.

Remember:

- all containers and suicide notes should be sent with the casualty to hospital
- record the names of substances taken

- contact the Poisons Information Centre for specific advice on management
- any vomitus should be sent with the casualty to hospital.

Poisons Information Centres

(Principal centres in each State and Territory. For further information, see any Telecom Australia directory.)

	STD Code	Telephone
Australian Capital Territory		
Royal Canberra Hospital	06	243 2154
New South Wales		
Royal Alexandra Hospital for Children	02	519 0466
24-hour, toll-free number	008	25 1525
Northern Territory		
Royal Darwin Hospital	089	22 8842
Queensland		
Brisbane Royal Children's Hospital	07	253 8233
For callers outside Brisbane	008	17 7333
South Australia		
Adelaide Children's Hospital	08	204 6117
For callers outside Adelaide	008	18 2111
Tasmania		
Royal Hobart Hospital	002	38 8485
For callers in Tasmania outside Hobart	008	00 1400
Victoria		
Royal Children's Hospital	03	345 5678
For callers outside Melbourne	008	13 3890
Western Australia		
Princess Margaret Hospital for Children	09	381 1177
For callers outside Perth	008	11 9244

Symptoms and signs

The symptoms and signs of poisoning depend on the nature of the intoxicating substance. Any of the following may occur:

- abdominal pain
- nausea and/or vomiting
- drowsiness
- burning pains, from the mouth to the stomach
- breathing difficulty
- tight chest
- headache
- ringing in the ears
- blurred vision
- a smell of fumes
- odours on the breath
- bite or injection marks, with or without local swelling
- contamination of the skin
- change of skin colour, with blueness of the lips
- burns around and inside the mouth, and to the tongue
- sudden collapse

Management — general rules

If the casualty is unconscious:

- □ DRABC
- □ call the Fire Brigade if the atmosphere is contaminated with smoke, gases, ammonia, etc.
- □ seek medical aid urgently.

If the casualty is conscious but uncooperative:
- □ listen to the casualty but do not give advice
- □ seek medical aid urgently.

If the casualty is conscious and cooperative:
- □ determine whether the substance is corrosive, petroleum-based, medicinal or a general substance
- □ manage according to the type of substance.

For a **swallowed corrosive or petroleum based** substance, e.g. dishwasher powder, toilet cleaner, kerosene, petrol:

- □ DRABC
- □ do not induce vomiting

☐ wash corrosive substance off mouth and face with water
☐ if within ten minutes after swallowing, give a small drink of milk or water; otherwise, give nothing by mouth
☐ seek medical aid urgently.

For a **swallowed medicinal or general** substance, e.g. detergent, medicine, mushrooms:
☐ DRABC
☐ induce vomiting by giving Syrup of Ipecac to drink, according to the instructions on the bottle. Do not give salt or soapy water to drink
☐ keep the casualty comfortable
☐ keep a sample of vomitus (about 100 millilitres) in a covered jar to be sent with casualty to hospital
☐ seek medical aid urgently.

For an **unknown** substance:
☐ DRABC
☐ do not induce vomiting
☐ seek medical aid urgently.

For **cyanide** (there may be a smell of 'bitter almonds'):
☐ DRABC
☐ turn the casualty on the side
☐ if breathing stops, wash the casualty's mouth and lips, and commence EAR. Do not inhale the casualty's expired air
☐ seek medical aid urgently.

For an **inhaled** substance:
☐ DRABC
☐ if necessary move the casualty to fresh air, taking care not to become the next casualty
☐ loosen tight clothing
☐ if the casualty has difficulty breathing or shows signs of intoxication, seek medical aid urgently.

For an **absorbed** substance:

DRABC

□ DRABC
□ ask the casualty to remove all clothing and shower the skin clean
□ ensure that contaminated clothes are laundered separately
□ if any symptoms and signs of poisoning are observed, seek medical aid.

16

Bites and stings

Bites and stings of some animals are potentially dangerous as a result of the venom which is injected or because the casualty is allergic to some insects.

Allergic reactions to insect bites

If the casualty has an allergic history or any signs of allergy, e.g. a rash, raised lumps on the skin, swelling of the throat, wheezing, manage as follows:

1 DRABC.

2 Apply pressure immobilization.

3 Seek medical aid urgently.

4 Periodically observe and record the pulse and breathing.

5 If the casualty is carrying any medication for the allergy, it should be taken at once. If the medication is not identified for this purpose (by the casualty, a relative, or the label), it should not be taken.

6 Carry out EAR or CPR if necessary.

Pressure immobilization is used in the case of an allergic reaction, or for management of bites and stings of the following:
- blue-ringed octopus
- box jellyfish
- cone shell
- funnel web spider
- snakes.

Pressure immobilization

Apply pressure immobilization over the bitten area and around the limb, using a crepe or conforming bandage about 15 cm wide. If unavailable, use pantyhose or other material.

1 Apply the bandage firmly enough to compress tissue, but not so firmly as to restrict the flow of blood to the limb below the bandage.

2 Bandage from the bite to the fingers or toes, then up to the armpit or groin.

3 Bandage as much of the limb as possible.

4 Apply a splint to the bandaged limb with a second bandage.

5 Do not remove the splint or bandage, once applied.

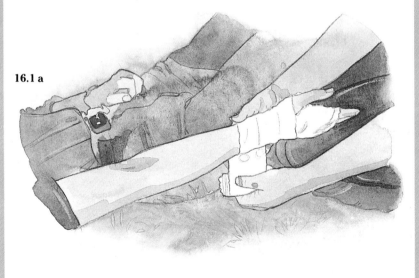

16.1 a

CONTINUED

CONTINUED

Pressure immobilization

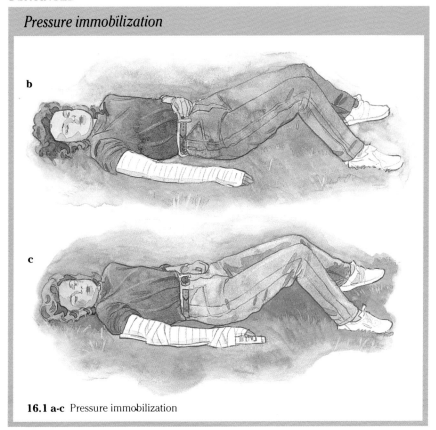

b

c

16.1 a-c Pressure immobilization

As a general rule, non-lethal bites and stings of land dwelling insects are managed by application of ice compresses, e.g.
- bee
- centipede
- European wasp
- red back spider
- scorpion.

Emergency first aid advice for marine stings is available from the Marine Stinger Reporting Service by phoning 008–079 909.

Detailed management of bites and stings of various animals and insects is described in the following alphabetical listing.

Bee

Bee stings are usually left behind in the skin with the venom sac attached.

Management

- remove sting by scraping it sideways with a fingernail or the side of a knife blade
- wipe the area clean
- apply cold compresses
- if there are signs of allergy, or if the casualty has an allergic history, see the section on allergic reactions at the beginning of this chapter.

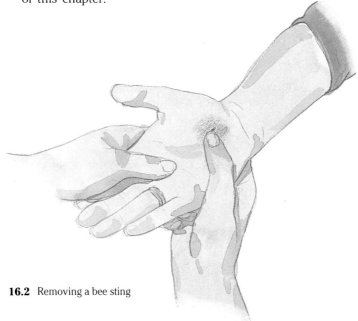

16.2 Removing a bee sting

Blue-ringed octopus

The bite of the blue-ringed octopus is normally painless so the casualty may be unaware of the danger.

Symptoms and signs

- swallowing difficulty
- blurred vision
- within minutes, numbness of the lips and tongue
- no breathing.

Management

- □ DRABC
- □ reassure the casualty and have him lie down
- □ as breathing difficulty progresses, commence EAR
- □ pressure immobilization
- □ seek medical aid urgently.

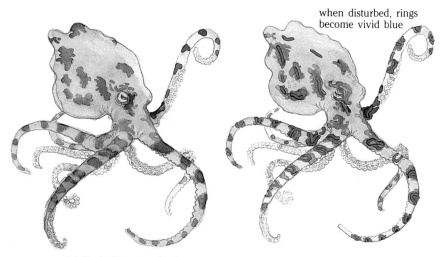

when disturbed, rings become vivid blue

16.3 a-b Blue-ringed octopus

Box jellyfish

Box jellyfish are normally found in tropical waters, from the Gladstone area in Queensland, north around the coast to Broome in Western Australia.

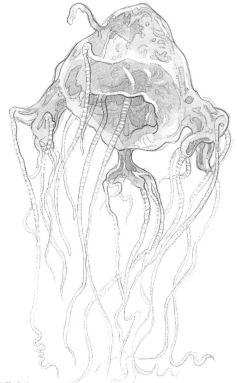

16.4 Box jellyfish

Prevention

- obey the instructions of surf lifesavers, particularly if they ask you to leave the water

- swim in stinger-resistant enclosures whenever possible
- wear protective clothing, e.g. a lycra stinger suit, or two pairs of pantyhose, one pair worn over the legs and abdomen, the other, with a small cut across the crotch, over the arms and chest, whenever swimming in tropical waters (even in enclosures) from October to May
- enter the water slowly — do not run or dive in
- if any sting is felt, back out of the water slowly. Do not struggle
- carry 4 litres of household vinegar and broad conforming or crepe bandages whenever you go to a tropical Australian beach
- if rescuing a casualty from the water, take care not to be stung.

Symptoms and signs

- immediate intense pain
- very obvious whip-like tentacle marks (deep red/mauve skin welts)
- characteristic 'frosted ladder' pattern may be visible
- breathing and circulation difficulties, with cessation of breathing sometimes within a few minutes
- casualty may be irrational. If he/she suddenly becomes quiet, check level of consciousness.

Management

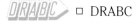

- ☐ DRABC
- ☐ **if necessary**, EAR or CPR
- ☐ do not rub the stung area
- ☐ if vinegar is available, flood the stung area for at least 30 seconds. Apply pressure immobilization over the area after flooding with vinegar. **Do not** cease resuscitation during this time

- if vinegar is not available, gently pick off any tentacles with tweezers or your fingers. Apply pressure immobilization only above the sting
- continually monitor breathing and circulation
- seek medical aid urgently
- immobilize bandaged limbs with splints and more bandages
- apply ice to relieve pain.

Bullrout

Bullrout are found in tropical inlets, rocky beaches, coral reefs and brackish estuaries.

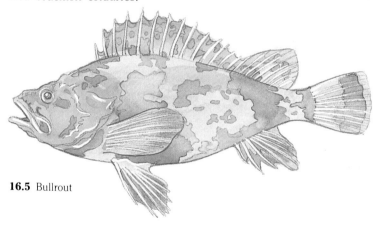

16.5 Bullrout

Prevention

- investigate before picking up 'funny looking rocks'
- take care when walking on rocks at the seaside. Always wear shoes
- do not put your hands or feet in rock crevices
- wear suitable footwear when wading in deep water or on mud flats.

Symptoms and signs

- immediate intense pain at the site of the puncture
- spread of pain along the limb
- sometimes, the presence of the stinging spine in the wound
- swelling
- stung area may be grey or blue
- the casualty may be irrational
- sometimes sweating and shock.

Management

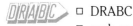

- ☐ DRABC
- ☐ seek medical aid urgently
- ☐ while waiting, place the affected part in hot fluids, e.g.water or hot drinks, for at least 20 minutes, being careful not to scald the casualty
- ☐ remove any foreign body that comes away easily
- ☐ reassure the casualty
- ☐ observe breathing, and be prepared to supplement the casualty's breathing with EAR if necessary.

Centipede

Centipede bites are painful but not normally dangerous.

Symptoms and signs

- immediate intense burning pain
- throbbing and later, numbness.

Management

- ☐ apply a cold pack or compress over the affected area
- ☐ seek medical aid.

Chironex box jellyfish

See box jellyfish.

Cone shell

Cone shell envenomation is normally painless so the casualty may be unaware of the danger.

For information on symptoms and signs, and management procedures, see section on blue-ringed octopus.

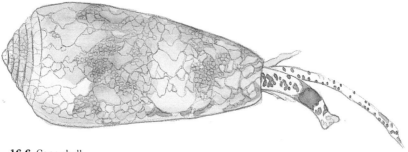

16.6 Cone shell

European wasp

The European wasp can sting several times, because unlike the bee, it does not leave its sting behind in the skin. It is attracted to meat that is being cooked, sweet drinks and decaying food.

Symptoms and signs

- extreme pain
- possibly swelling and blockage of the airway, resulting in breathing difficulty, if stung in the mouth.

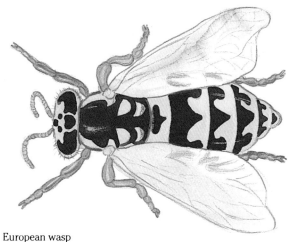

16.7 European wasp

Management

☐ DRABC (give EAR if necessary)
☐ wash the area clean
☐ apply cold compresses
☐ if there are signs of allergy, or if the casualty has a history of allergy, see the section on allergic reactions at the beginning of this chapter.

Funnel web spider

The funnel web spider is found around Sydney, on the New South Wales coast and in south-east Queensland. It is a large black or reddish-brown spider, 2 or 3 cm in length.
It is found:

- in rock crevices
- in burrows
- in post holes
- underneath houses
- in trees and shrubs.

Prevention

- show children pictures of the spider and tell them to leave such spiders alone
- if living in areas known to be infested, clean out obvious habitats.

Symptoms and signs

- initially, intense pain at the site of the bite
- nausea and abdominal pain
- breathing may be difficult and noisy
- numbness
- muscular weakness
- profuse sweating
- saliva from the mouth
- coughing up of secretions
- weeping from the eyes
- cold skin and shivering.

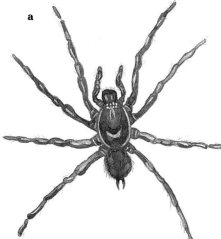
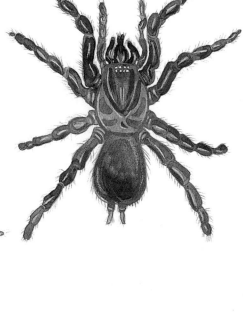

16.8 a-b Funnel web spider

Management

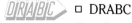

- □ DRABC
- □ rest and reassure casualty
- □ apply a pressure immobilization bandage over the bitten area and around the limb
- □ seek medical aid urgently.

Jellyfish

For symptoms and signs, and management procedures for box jellyfish stings, see box jellyfish. The following information relates to jellyfish, e.g. bluebottles, which are common in Australian oceans.

Symptoms and signs

- visual evidence of stinging, e.g. weals, whip marks, localized area of goose pimples
- pain in the stung area
- pain in the chest and abdomen
- backache
- nausea and/or vomiting
- lack of coordination in the limbs
- breathing difficulty, 10 to 40 minutes after stinging.

Management

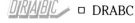

- □ DRABC
- □ reassure the casualty
- □ if any tentacles remain, gently pick off with tweezers or your fingers, or wash off with water
- □ apply cold packs or crushed ice wrapped in a thin towel or cloth to the stung area. Continue until pain is relieved

◻ do not rub the area
◻ restrain the casualty's hands
◻ seek medical aid.

Lizards

Lizards may bite if handled. The bite is not venomous but may become infected.
● if the lizard will not let go, apply a lighted match to its mouth
● manage the wound
● seek medical aid.

Red back spider

The red back spider is small, normally black with a red stripe on the back.

It is found:
● throughout most parts of Australia
● in dark, unattended spots, e.g. under eaves, in old tyres, in garden sheds.

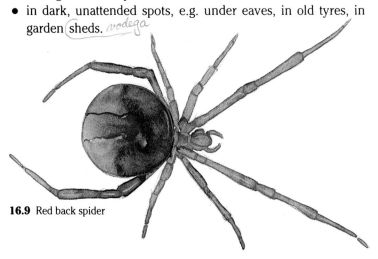

16.9 Red back spider

Prevention

- clean out habitats and treat the area with a suitable pesticide
- use gloves when handling old tyres, cleaning out sheds, or carrying out other tasks likely to involve contact with the red back spider.

Symptoms and signs

- a sharp sting may be felt
- pain at the site of the bite, which then becomes general
- nausea
- dizziness and sometimes faintness
- muscle weakness or spasm
- sweating, sometimes profuse
- swelling and localized sweating around the bite
- rapid pulse.

Management

- ☐ DRABC
- ☐ reassure the casualty
- ☐ apply a cold pack or compress over the area
- ☐ seek medical aid.

Scorpion

For information on symptoms and signs, and management procedures, see section on centipedes.

Snakes

Snakes are not normally aggressive and tend to bite only when they are threatened or mishandled. Some snakes, e.g. the carpet snake, are not venomous. Others, e.g. the brown snake, tiger snake and taipan, are very poisonous.

Prevention

- leave snakes alone and do not collect snakes
- in snake infested country, wear stout shoes, walk-socks and jeans or similar clothing
- do not wear sandals or thongs or walk in bare feet in places where snakes could be present
- do not put your hands in hollow logs, under piles of wood, or in rubbish
- be noisy when walking in the bush
- look carefully when walking through thick grass
- use a torch around camps or farm houses at night
- keep sheds free of mice
- cut grass short around houses and in school playgrounds.

Symptoms and signs

These do not appear immediately, but from about 15 minutes to 2 hours after the casualty is bitten. There are often no visible symptoms and signs. Take seriously any information that a casualty has been bitten by a snake:

- strong emotional reaction
- headache
- double vision
- drowsiness
- nausea and/or vomiting and diarrhoea
- pain or tightness in the chest or abdomen

- giddiness or faintness
- puncture marks about 1 centimetre apart at the site of the bite, although sometimes there may only be fang scratches on the skin. Bites are usually on the limbs, especially the legs
- swelling of the bitten area
- reddening
- bruising
- sweating
- breathing difficulties.

Management

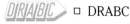

- ☐ DRABC
- ☐ rest and reassure the casualty
- ☐ apply a pressure immobilization bandage over the bitten area and around the limb (see section on pressure immobilization at the beginning of this chapter)
- ☐ seek medical aid urgently.

a

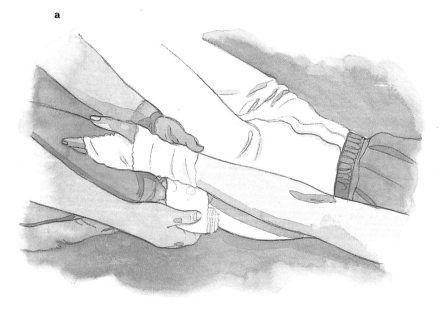

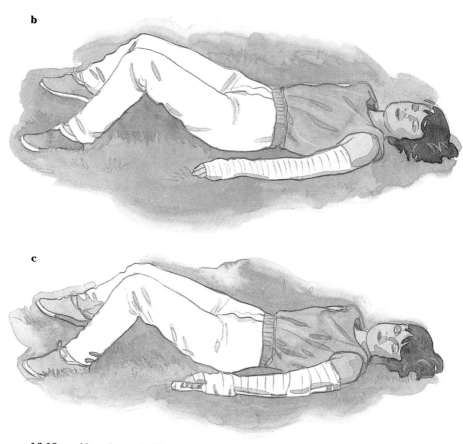

16.10 a-c Managing snake bite

Warning:

- **never** wash the venom off the skin as this will help in later identification
- **never** cut or excise the bitten area
- **never** try to suck the venom out of the wound
- **never** use a constrictive bandage
- **do not** try to catch the snake. However, a description of the snake may assist medical aid.

Sting ray

The sting is attached half way along the sting ray's whip-like tail. This can inflict a very painful wound.

Prevention

- when wading in shallow water, wear protective footwear and shuffle.

Symptoms and signs

- immediate intense burning pain
- possible breathing difficulty
- bleeding from the wound.

Management

- ☐ DRABC
- ☐ gently extract the barb if visible
- ☐ bathe with hot water, being careful to test for tolerance temperature with an **uninjured** limb as the stung area may be partly anaesthetized from the toxin
- ☐ seek medical aid.

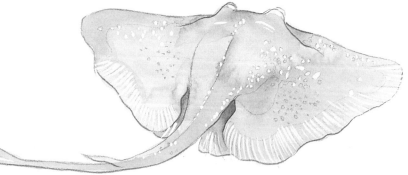

16.11 Sting ray

Stonefish

Stonefish are found in tropical inlets, rocky beaches, coral reefs and brackish estuaries. For information and symptoms and signs and management procedures, see bullrout.

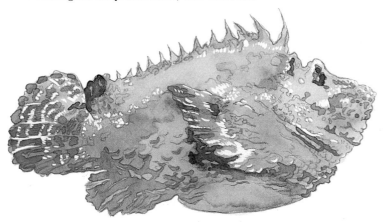

16.12 Stonefish

Ticks

Ticks occur in most parts of Australia. However, paralysis ticks occur mainly along coastal eastern Australia, from Queensland to northern Tasmania. Usually drab in colour, ticks are oval and flat. Engorged, they may become globular and about 0.5 centimetres in diameter. They may hide in body crevices. The venom may cause paralysis, especially in small children. Many ticks do not cause paralysis, but may cause local irritation or a skin nodule.

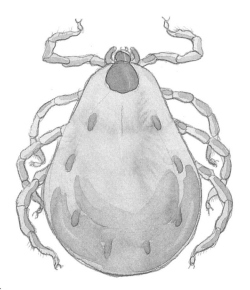

16.13 Tick

Symptoms and signs

- weakness of the face and upper eyelids, progressing to arms and breathing muscles.

Management

☐ if in the ear, seek medical aid

☐ remove the tick by sliding the open blades of a pair of small sharp scissors or tweezers, one each side of the tick, and lever the tick outwards, being careful not to leave the mouth parts in the skin

☐ search carefully for other ticks, particularly in the hair, behind the ears and other body crevices

☐ if the casualty does not recover after a few hours or if the casualty is a child, seek medical aid.

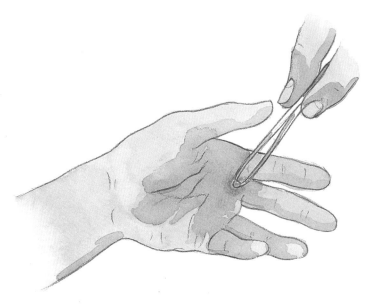

16.14 Removing a tick

17

Over-exposure to heat and cold

Overexposure to heat

The temperature of the healthy human body is maintained at about 37°C. In hot or humid conditions, e.g. in a boiler room, or travelling in hot climates, people are at risk of heat illness.

There are three stages of heat illness:
- heat cramps *calambres*
- heat exhaustion
- heat stroke.

Prevention

- protect yourself from strong direct sunlight
- wear loose fitting porous clothing and a broad brimmed hat
- do not do heavy physical tasks in hot humid weather unless conditioned to the task and the environmental conditions
- drink enough water to satisfy your thirst
- avoid alcohol, as this increases urine output, and hence fluid loss
- do not spend prolonged periods in saunas
- do not leave infants or children in closed cars during hot weather
- cease working when affected by heat cramps or heat exhaustion and seek medical aid if the symptoms persist
- do not take part in 'fun runs' and similar activities during the hot summer months.

Heat cramps

Symptoms and signs

- painful muscle cramps of the limbs and abdomen, either while resting or exercising
- nausea and/or vomiting

- tiredness, dizziness or weakness
- moist cool skin.

Management

☐ remove the casualty to a cool place, if possible
☐ have the casualty lie down
☐ replace lost fluid by giving plenty of water to which may be added glucose or sugar. If commercial preparations are used, they should be diluted as recommended by the manufacturer. If the casualty is nauseated, encourage slow drinking
☐ apply ice packs to the cramped muscles
☐ gently stretch the muscles, but do not massage
☐ warn the casualty that further exertion and exposure in the hot environment may lead to heat exhaustion and that he/she should rest or work in a cooler area and/or at a less physically demanding task.

Heat exhaustion

Heat exhaustion occurs mostly in hot, humid climates. The young and the elderly are more at risk, as are dehydrated casualties and those wearing unsuitable clothing when working or exercising.

Symptoms and signs

- feeling hot, exhausted and weak, with a headache which may have persisted for some hours or days
- thirst
- fatigue
- nausea
- loss of appetite
- giddiness and faintness

- stomach and muscle cramps
- shortness of breath
- muscular weakness
- lack of coordination
- pale, cool and clammy skin
- profuse sweating
- rapid breathing and pulse
- possibly, confusion or irritability.

Management

- □ move the casualty to a cool place with circulating air, and lay him/her down
- □ loosen any tight clothing and remove any unnecessary garments
- □ sponge the body down with cold water, but do not overcool
- □ replace lost fluid (as for management of heat cramps)
- □ seek medical aid if the casualty vomits and cannot keep fluid down, or does not recover promptly
- □ manage cramps as previously outlined.

Heat stroke

Heat stroke is a potentially lethal condition. Early recognition of heat stroke is essential. Those at risk of heat stroke include:
- infants left in closed cars on a hot day
- athletes attempting to run long distances in hot weather, particularly fun runners
- unfit workers and overweight alcoholics in hot climates
- the elderly or ill.

Symptoms and signs

- headache
- nausea and/or vomiting

- dizziness
- visual disturbances
- often, irritability or mental confusion, and possibly aggression
- altered mental state, which may progress to seizures and unconsciousness
- a rise in body temperature to 40°C or more
- a strong pounding and rapid pulse
- skin flushed, and usually dry.

Management

☐ DRABC
☐ remove the casualty to a cool place
☐ loosen any tight clothing and remove any unnecessary garments

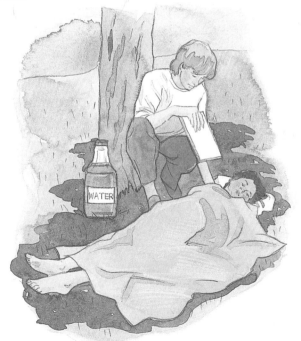

17.1 Managing heat stroke

□ apply cold packs or ice to the areas of large blood vessels, such as the neck, groin and armpits, to accelerate cooling

□ if possible, cover the casualty's body with a wet sheet and fan to increase air circulation

□ continue until the body feels cold to the touch, then stop cooling

□ seek medical aid urgently

□ when the casualty is fully conscious give fluids, e.g. water to which is added glucose and salt (as for management of heat cramps).

Overexposure to cold

Overexposure to cold can occur:
- following immersion
- as a result of wind chill
- when in the snow without protective clothing
- in lightly clad runners and motorcyclists exposed to wind
- in divers
- in unconscious, immobile or drugged persons in a cold environment
- in young children, babies and the elderly in a cold environment.

The severity of overexposure depends on:
- age and physical condition
- clothing
- temperature
- wind speed
- period of exposure

The following will accelerate the condition:
- low atmospheric temperature

- wind, snow, rain
- fatigue
- anxiety
- hunger.

Prevention

- wear warm inner clothing made from material specially designed for extremely cold environments
- wear wind and waterproof outer clothing
- ensure adequate protection of the ears and nose
- have a minimum of four persons in your party
- ask locals about usual weather conditions if boating, skiing or mountain climbing in an unfamiliar area
- listen to broadcast weather reports
- be sure that boats or other equipment are in good condition
- have adequate sleeping bags and covers
- eat adequate food before departure
- take adequate food and drink (not alcohol) with you
- inform people of your departure and expected time of return
- if caught in bad weather take shelter early and watch for signs of cold exposure
- take steps to avoid more physical activity than is necessary when conditions are extremely cold.

Mild to moderate overexposure to cold

Symptoms and signs

- a cold feeling and shivering
- excessive fatigue
- problems with vision
- faintness
- cramps

- increasing slowness of physical and mental responses
- uncoordinated movement, e.g. stumbling
- confusion
- slurred speech.

Management

- □ DRABC
- □ protect the casualty and yourself from wind, rain and sleet and from cold, wet ground
- □ if possible, remove wet clothing and wrap the casualty in warm, dry clothing or a space blanket

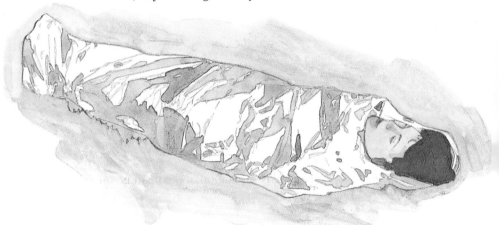

17.2 Managing overexposure to cold

- □ if possible, put the casualty in a warmed sleeping bag
- □ if the casualty is conscious give warm fluids to drink
- □ do not give alcohol
- □ place the casualty in a bath of water heated to about 37°C and raise the temperature of the bathwater slowly to about 40°C.
- □ if a warm bath is not available, a companion stripped to underclothing and sharing the casualty's sleeping bag can help to warm the body

□ do not try to warm the casualty in front of a fire
□ seek medical aid if recovery is not prompt
□ remain with the casualty until medical aid arrives.

Severe accidental cooling (hypothermia)

Hypothermia is a dangerous condition, commonly caused by prolonged immersion in cold water. Infants, the infirm and the elderly are especially at risk. Alcohol, drugs and injury may aggravate the condition.

Symptoms and signs

- coldness
- slow pulse
- slow, shallow breathing
- quietness and refusal of food in infants
- unconsciousness, especially in the elderly or the ill.

Management

□ DRABC — it is important to ensure that breathing and pulse are absent before commencing resuscitation. If the heart is still beating, even slowly, commencing resuscitation could be lethal.
□ remove to a warm dry place if possible
□ place the casualty between blankets so that the temperature can rise gradually
□ if conscious, give warm drinks (not alcohol)
□ a companion stripped to underclothing and sharing the casualty's sleeping bag can help to warm the body
□ seek medical aid urgently
□ remain with the casualty until medical aid arrives.

Warning: do not attempt to speed up the warming process by placing the casualty in a hot bath, or by using hot water bottles or electric blankets.

Frostbite

Frostbite results in local freezing of body tissue, e.g. toes, fingers and other extremities. Deep frostbite may affect the blood supply so badly that amputation may be necessary.

Superficial frostbite

Symptoms and signs

- numbness and tingling in exposed areas
- sudden whiteness of the skin
- waxy appearance
- firmness to touch
- area is painless until rewarmed
- possible blistering.

Management

- ☐ remove the casualty to a warm dry place
- ☐ remove anything constricting the affected limb
- ☐ rewarm the area by body heat
- ☐ never rub or massage the frostbitten area
- ☐ never apply snow or cold water
- ☐ never rewarm with direct heat
- ☐ cover any blisters with dry sterile dressings
- ☐ give no alcohol
- ☐ seek medical aid.

Deep frostbite

Symptoms and signs

In addition to those for superficial frostbite:
- the area is white, hard to the touch and painless.

Management

- □ do not attempt to thaw
- □ keep the casualty dry and warm
- □ protect the injured area from further injury
- □ seek medical aid urgently.

Cold metal injury

Wear gloves to avoid skin adhering to extremely cold metal.

Management

- □ pour warm water over the part, and when free, manage as for superficial frostbite
- □ seek medical aid for blistering or other tissue damage.

18

Traffic accident injuries

Danger

- ensure that you, others and the casualty are safe
- avoid danger from oncoming traffic. Protect the scene by parking your car between it and approaching traffic
- switch on hazard warning lights or indicators
- station people to warn other motorists of the accident, particularly if the scene is not visible to approaching vehicles
- at night, light up the scene with headlights on low beam
- set up reflective warning triangles if available
- keep clear of fallen electricity wires
- ensure that all occupants of the vehicle(s) are accounted for
- check for the presence of flammable liquids, e.g. petrol, and if possible, have fire extinguishers ready for use
- casualties may be trapped and injuries may be hidden by wreckage
- turn off the ignition of the crashed vehicle, apply the handbrake and chock wheels if on a slope
- protect the casualty from battery acid, hot liquids, engine or exhaust parts
- do not disconnect the battery of a damaged vehicle.

Do not:

- smash glass unless the casualty is protected
- attempt to right an overturned vehicle
- allow smoking at the scene of an accident
- touch the vehicle or occupants if fallen electricity wires are in contact with the vehicle.

Calling help

- dial 000 in any state capital, or the number listed in the telephone directory. If another vehicle has CB radio, use it to call help
- instruct a bystander to contact the nearest ambulance or emergency service and police
- **ensure that the message is understood**
- check the approximate waiting time before help will arrive.

Helping the trapped casualty

- DRABC
- send for expert assistance urgently
- if the door nearest the casualty is jammed, try to gain entry through other doors or windows
- if possible, remove heavy objects. If the dashboard or steering wheel are compressing the casualty's chest, slide the seat back or tilt the back of the seat down slightly
- tilt the casualty's head backwards, with jaw support so that the airway remains open

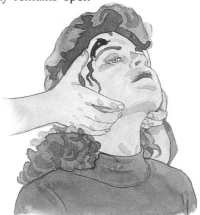

18.1 Opening the airway of a trapped casualty

- look under debris in the vehicle to ensure that no casualties are hidden from view
- ensure that battery acid, hot water, oil or petrol do not splash onto the casualty
- **do not** remove the casualty, particularly if unconscious, unless absolutely necessary. Wait for expert help.

Dangerous situations where you may need to move a casualty from inside a crashed vehicle

1 When there is evidence of increasing shock and the casualty is upright in the car.

2 When the casualty is unconscious and an adequate airway cannot be maintained.

3 When the casualty's position prevents access to control bleeding.

4 When there is danger of fire.

Moving a casualty from inside a crashed vehicle

- DRABC
- only remove the casualty if in danger, as described above
- keep the airway clear
- try to support the spine and head in such a way as to avoid movement in any direction
- apply a cervical collar while the casualty is still in the vehicle
- recruit enough people to support all parts of the casualty's body
- give your helpers clear instructions on how the casualty is to be moved
- carry out the movement smoothly.

Moving a casualty from beneath a vehicle

If a casualty is trapped under a vehicle and has to be moved before expert help arrives, the vehicle may need to be raised:

- DRABC
- chock the wheels and use packing, e.g. blocks of timber, as the vehicle is raised. Raise only to a level that enables you to free the casualty
- move the casualty as gently as possible, supporting the head and neck
- when removing a casualty from beneath a motorcycle, avoid handling hot engine and exhaust parts
- note the exact position of the casualty and vehicle before moving, for reporting to police.

Motorcyclists' protective helmets

Only remove a helmet if absolutely necessary, e.g. when it is obstructing the casualty's breathing or if the casualty is vomiting. If removal is necessary, ask the casualty to remove it if possible.

To remove an open face helmet:
- unfasten or cut through the chin strap
- force the sides apart

18.2 a

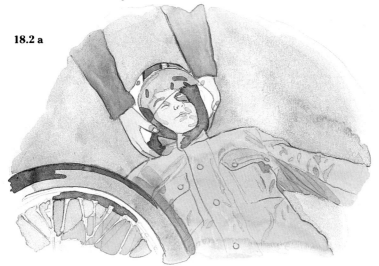

- lift the helmet upwards and backwards.

b

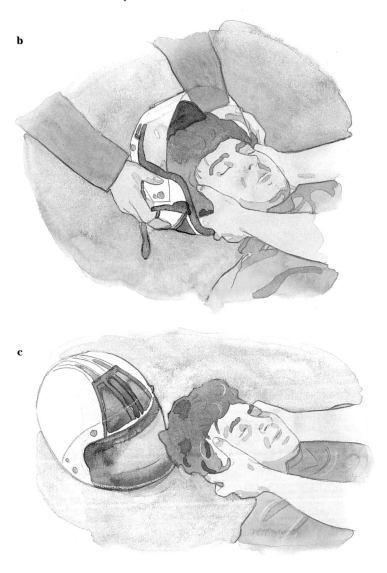

c

18.2 a-c Removing a motorcyclist's helmet (open face)

To remove a full face helmet:
- unfasten or cut through the chin strap
- one person must support the casualty's head and neck while the other lifts the helmet
- tilt the helmet back

18.3 a

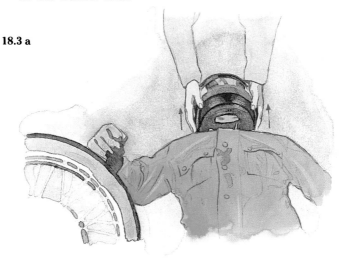

- lift it clear of the chin

b

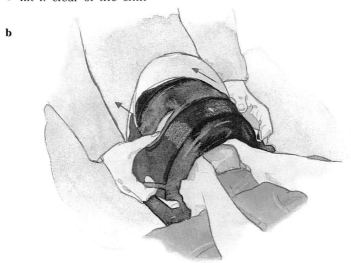

- tilt it slowly forward to pass over the base of the skull.

c

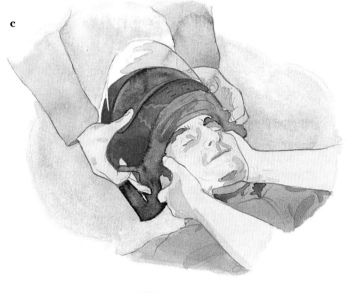

d

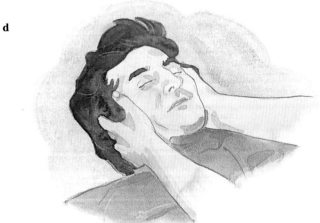

18.3 a-d Removing a motorcyclist's helmet (full face)

19

Communicable diseases and the first aider

Communicable diseases are those diseases which can be spread from one person to another. They are caused by germs such as bacteria and viruses.

Medical studies have indicated that a first aider is unlikely to develop any of these diseases as a result of attending to a casualty. Because the risk to the first aider is so low, it is advised that first aid should not be withheld.

Many communicable diseases can be present in the body before symptoms and signs become evident. Therefore the first aider should assume that any casualty may provide an element of risk, and should always observe hygiene procedures, as described in this chapter.

Some illnesses that may result, in either rescuer or casualty, from contact during resuscitation procedures

- colds
- influenza
- measles and mumps
- glandular fever
- hepatitis strains
- HIV infection
- herpes
- tuberculosis
- some forms of meningitis
- some skin infections, e.g. impetigo.

These diseases may be passed on by some of the following

- by blood and body fluids, e.g. saliva, vomit, pus, urine, seminal fluid, vaginal fluid, faeces and possibly breast milk

- by infected hypodermic needles or sharp objects
- through sexual intercourse where one partner is infected
- by sharing hypodermic needles that have been used by/on an infected person
- through transfusions of contaminated blood or injections of contaminated blood products
- through droplet infection
- an infected mother can pass diseases to her child before and during birth, or possibly through breast milk.

First aiders need to be careful to avoid contamination through cuts, grazes or mucous membranes, or from infected hypodermic needles or sharp objects that may pierce the skin.

Steps to take before management of a casualty

Use the following checklist of hygiene procedures before managing a casualty:
- wash your hands thoroughly with soap and water if available
- cover exposed cuts and grazes with waterproof dressings
- put on disposable plastic or rubber gloves, if available. These should be long enough to cover the lower forearms and/or to be tucked under the sleeves
- put on a plastic apron to protect clothes, if available.

Hygiene after management

Use the following checklist of hygiene procedures after managing a casualty:
- if clothing has been splashed with blood or body fluids, it is advisable to soak it in the strongest recommended solution of a name-brand household bleach for 30 minutes. Usually this solution will be one part of bleach to nine parts of water, but you should follow the instructions on the container. Always

use a freshly prepared solution of bleach. Wash clothing following disinfection. If bleaching is not appropriate, machine-wash clothing in the normal way, using the hottest possible water temperature

- clean contaminated surfaces by covering for 30 minutes with paper towels which have been soaked in the strongest recommended solution of a name-brand household bleach. Wash the wet areas with water and household detergent, and dry them thoroughly
- burn combustible waste materials
- waste materials that cannot be burned should be placed in a plastic bag inside another plastic bag. Tie the bags securely and dispose of them safely. Seek advice about safe disposal from your local hospital or doctor
- if a mask is used for resuscitation, wash it thoroughly in cold running tap water, making sure that no splashing of nearby areas occurs. Soak the mask for 30 minutes in the strongest recommended solution of a name-brand household bleach. Wash it thoroughly in water and household detergent and dry well
- finally, wash your hands thoroughly with soap and water.

Remember:

- if splashed by blood or other body fluids, skin should be washed thoroughly with soap and running tap water
- if lips, mouth, tongue, eyes or broken skin come into contact with blood or other body fluids, wash thoroughly with clean, cold running tap water
- if skin is punctured by a sharp object that may be contaminated, wash the area thoroughly with soap and running tap water, and seek medical advice as soon as possible
- use household bleach only in well ventilated areas
- do not put plastic bags of non-combustible waste material in the rubbish tin.

Recommended equipment

St John Ambulance Australia has prepared a Communicable Diseases Protection Pack to be used in conjunction with first aid kits. It contains a face mask, disposable goggles and gloves.

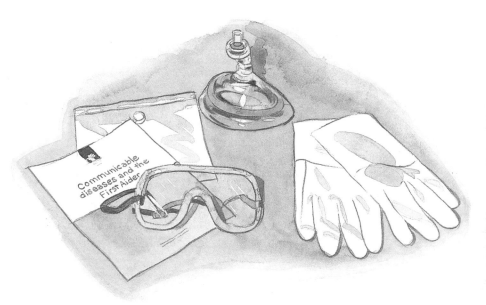

19.1 Communicable Diseases Protection Pack

Glossary

Abdomen	part of the body between the chest and the pelvis, containing digestive organs
Abrasion	an open wound caused by direct contact with a rough surface
Absent breathing	no perceptible sign of breathing
Absent circulation	no perceptible pulse
Absent pulse	no detectable heartbeat
Absorb	to take up fluids or gases
Acetone	a colourless liquid which is used as a solvent and smells like nail polish remover
Acid	a corrosive substance; a neutralizer of an alkali
Acute pain	pain which is sharp, severe and short in duration
Airway	the passage by which air enters and leaves the lungs
Alkali	a corrosive substance; a neutralizer of acid
Allergic	sensitive to some substance, such as bee venom
Amputation	the cutting off of a limb, digit, or appendage

Angina pectoris	a heart condition in which there is an acute pain in the chest caused by interference with the supply of oxygen to the heart, usually brought on by exercise or anxiety
Antiseptic	a substance that helps to prevent the growth of germs
Anus	the external opening of the rectum
Artery	a vessel carrying blood away from the heart
Asphyxia	lack of oxygen and increase of carbon dioxide in the body
Assessment	evaluation of problems affecting the casualty as indicated by the history, symptoms and signs observed by the first aider
Asthma	spasm of the bronchial tubes
Bandage	material used to cover or hold in place a sterile dressing
Bowel	part of the digestive canal below the stomach and duodenum
Breastbone	the flat bone which forms the middle of the front of the chest and which separates the ribs
Capillaries	smallest blood vessels
Cardiopulmonary resuscitation	a resuscitation technique that combines expired air resuscitation with external cardiac compression
Carotid pulse	the heartbeat as felt in the arteries of the neck

Casualty	someone who has suffered an accident or sudden illness
Cervical	pertaining to the neck
Cholesterol	fatty substance deposited from the blood in the arteries
Circulation	the movement of blood through the body
Combustible	able to be burned
Communicable diseases	diseases, caused by germs such as bacteria and viruses, that can be spread from one person to another
Compress	a cold dressing that assists control of bruising and swelling, and helps relieve pain
Concussion	injury to the brain, usually caused by a blow, sometimes leading to dizziness, nausea, loss of consciousness and weak pulse
Constrictive bandage	a firmly applied bandage above the injury site, and above the middle joint of the limb, to control bleeding; used only when direct pressure fails
Convulsions	violent and involuntary contractions of the muscles, often called seizures or fits
Cornea	the 'window' of the eye
Corrosive	destroying gradually; eating away a surface
CPR	cardiopulmonary resuscitation
Crater wound	wound caused by tissue being torn from the body

DRABC	stands for Danger, Response, Airway, Breathing, Circulation — the St John Action Plan for first aid management
Dehydration	excessive loss of salt and water from the body
Diabetes	disease of the insulin-producing cells in the pancreas
Diaphragm	the dome-shaped muscular wall separating the abdomen from the chest cavity
Direct pressure	method for controlling bleeding
Disc	a layer of fibro-elastic tissue between two vertebrae
Dislocation	injuries in which the bones of a joint are pushed out of normal contact with each other
Disorientation	a state of mental confusion, particularly relating to time and place
Distend	swell out, inflate
EAR	expired air resuscitation
ECC	external cardiac compression
Envenomation	poisoning from bites, stings or penetrating wounds — usually from reptiles, insects and marine creatures
Epilepsy	a condition of the brain leading to seizures
Exhale	breathe out
Expired air resuscitation	the technique used by the first aider when the casualty is unable to breathe. Also known as EAR

External cardiac compression	compression of the heart from outside the body by pressing on the breastbone in order to try to provide artificial circulation of the blood
Extremities	fingers and toes
Faeces	waste food products passed by the bowel
Fainting	a form of loss of consciousness
Flail chest	a condition caused by multiple fractures of the ribs and instability of the rib cage
Flammable	easily set on fire
Forearm	the part of the arm between the elbow and the wrist
Fracture	a break in a bone
Genitals	the reproductive organs
Heart	the hollow muscular organ responsible for pumping blood
Heat stroke	a serious, life-threatening condition in which the body's temperature is dangerously high
History	when relating to first aid, the story of the incident or the illness obtained from the casualty or witnesses
Hyperglycaemia	high blood sugar
Hypoglycaemia	low blood sugar
Hypothermia	the severe accidental cooling of the body
Immobilize	to prevent from moving
Incision	a cut made by a sharp instrument

Infection	the invasion and growth of harmful germs in the tissues of the body
Inflammable	easily set on fire
Inflammation	may be caused by infection and is characterized by pain, heat, swelling and redness
Inhale	breathe in
Insulin	a hormone produced in the pancreas which controls the use of sugar in the body
Intestines	the lower part of the alimentary canal
Intoxication	a state of excitement or drunkenness induced by alcohol or other drugs
Ipecacuanha	a drug used to induce vomiting, also known as Syrup of Ipecac
Irrigate	to wash a wound with a constant stream of water
Jaw support, jaw thrust	procedures for opening the airway
Lethal	deadly
Ligaments	tissues connecting bones at joints
Liver	a large organ located in the upper abdomen
Lungs	the pair of breathing organs in the chest cavity
Medication	medicine
Microorganisms	germs

Mucus	sticky fluid from some parts of the body, e.g. the nose, bronchi
Nausea	a feeling of sickness
Nerves	tissues that convey impulses from one part of the body to another
Nostril	the openings of the nose
Obstructed	blocked
Oxygen	a gaseous element of air that we breathe in
Pallor	paleness of skin
Pancreas	a gland that produces insulin and alkaline digestive matter
Paradoxical breathing	seen in flail chest injuries — the injured side moves in on inspiration and balloons out on expiration
Paralysis	loss or impairment of the ability to move parts of the body
Pelvis	the bone structure that forms the lowest part of the trunk
Posture	the body's attitude
Pressure pad	firm pad applied over dressing to assist in control of bleeding
Pressure points	points where pressure can be applied to control bleeding
Pulmonary	relating to the lungs
Pulse	the transmission of the heartbeat felt in various parts of the body

Pupil	the opening in the centre of the iris of the eye
Respiration	breathing
Response	the first aider's means of assessing the casualty's state of consciousness
Resuscitation	reviving one who is seriously injured or apparently dead
RICE	Rest, ice, compression, elevation: the method used by first aiders to manage soft tissue injuries
Saliva	secretions in the mouth
Seizures	violent muscular contraction and relaxation (convulsions)
Shock	a condition in which the circulatory system is not carrying sufficient blood to the tissues
Signs	the features of the casualty's condition that can be seen, felt, heard or smelt
Sinus	any of the eight cavities in the skull that are connected with the nasal cavity
Skeleton	bones of the body
Skull	the bony framework of the head, enclosing and protecting the brain, and consisting of the cranium and the facial section
Spasm	sudden involuntary muscular contraction
Spinal cord	the bundle of nervous tissue extending from the base of the brain and which is surrounded and protected by the spine

Spleen	an organ in the abdomen
Sprain	stretching of the ligaments
Sputum	mucus from the lungs, bronchi and throat that is ejected through the mouth
Sterile	free of germs
Strain	overstretching or overexertion of a muscle
Stroke	a cerebro-vascular accident resulting in partial paralysis
Suffocation	death from lack of oxygen
Symptoms	what the casualty tells you about his condition
Syrup of Ipecac	a drug used to induce vomiting
Tetanus	a serious and potentially fatal infection
Toxic	poisonous
Unconsciousness	a condition in which the brain fails to respond to the messages sent to it
Urine	waste products removed from the blood by the kidneys
Vagina	the passage leading inwards from the external female genitalia
Venom	a poison, normally from a snake, insect, marine creature or other animal
Vertebrae	(singular: vertebra) the individual bones that make up the spinal column
Vomitus	stomach contents vomited up

Index

Page numbers in italics refer to illustrations